The
Fitness
Instinct

The Fitness Instinct

The revolutionary
new approach to
healthy exercise
that is fun, natural,
and no sweat

PEG JORDAN

R.N., Editor and founder, *American Fitness* magazine

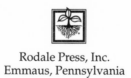

Rodale Press, Inc.
Emmaus, Pennsylvania

Printed in the United States of America on acid-free ∞, recycled paper ♻

Jacket and Interior Designer: Joanna Reinhart
Jacket Photographer: Tom Graves

Library of Congress Cataloging-in-Publication Data

Jordan, Peg.
    The fitness instinct : the revolutionary new approach to healthy exercise that is fun, natural, and no sweat / Peg Jordan.
      p.   cm.
    Includes index.
    ISBN 1–57954–005–8 hardcover
    1. Physical fitness.   2. Exercise.   I. Title.
    GV481.J694   1999
    613.7'1—dc21   99–34121

Distributed to the book trade by St. Martin's Press

2   4   6   8   10   9   7   5   3   hardcover

Visit us on the Web at www.rodalebooks.com, or call us toll-free at (800) 848-4735.

—— OUR PURPOSE ——

We inspire and enable people to improve their lives and the world around them.

In memory of George Sheehan, M.D., who taught me that fitness is more of a philosophy of spirit than a prescription of numbers.

acknowledgments

The Fitness Instinct was built on the best wishes of the most supportive network of family, friends, and colleagues anyone could hope for. My gratitude knows no bounds.

- For love of life: Claire, Adam, and Stu, and in honor of Mom and Dad
- For going forth confidently, with time to laugh: Mary Beth, Michelle, and Chrissy
- For believing in my ability to deliver the message long before I did: my agent and friend, Bonnie Solow
- For exquisite editing: Alisa Bauman, John Reeser, and my publisher at Rodale, Neil Wertheimer
- For being my best friend, unparalleled teaching, and continuous praise: Nancy Gillette
- For lessons in balance: Joel and Michelle Levey
- For lessons in motivating from the heart: Richard Simmons
- For their nods of approval and mastery: T. G. Harris, George Leonard, and Annie Styron
- For empowering friendship: Cheryl and Dean Radetsky, Tony Rich, Sidne Long, Melissa Johnson, Kate and Hilton, Judi Sheppard Misset, Cindy Schofield, Louise and Harvey, and Jeffrey Wattss
- For connecting and supporting: Linda Pfeffer, Beth Greer, Beverly Rubik, Steven Goldberg, Richard Gelb, John McCarthy, and Greg Angsten
- For pioneering work: Bill Hettler, Bud Getchell, Lauve Metcalf, Mary Guidron, Elaine and Joe Sullivan, Jack Travis, Mirka Knaster, Don Johnson, Tina Stromstead, Nancy Minges, Cynthia Borschetta, Suki Miller, Elisa Lodge, David Parker, and Paul Linden

- For mapping new territory: Linda Shelton, Marti West, Laura Gladwin, Gail Johnston, Susan Johnson, Mary Guidron, Kathie Davis, and Kristi Rudolph
- For Lake Louise camaraderie and new fitness vision: Neil Sol, Richard Keelor, Don Ardell, Brent Arnold, Ruth Alexander, Kirk Bauer, Don Chu, Laurie Kelley, George Pfeiffer, John Burstein, John Cates, Steve Ramirez, Don Powell, Charlie Kuntzleman, Doris McHugh, Sandy Trombetta, Gina Oliva, Joanne Owens-Nauslar, Joanie Sullivan-Morris, and Barb Harris
- For keeping the lights burning at NFLA and throughout our imaginations: Bob Karch
- For crone wisdom: Rita Lynne and Elinor Gadon
- For feminine sacred energy: Vicki Noble, Mara Keller, Rose Frances, Ani Mander, Z Budapest, and the crew at Esalen
- For all the students, clients, patients, and readers who have taught me everything I know about moving in harmony with your own heartbeat

contents

The Path
to Instinctual Fitness

Glistening hard-bodies strut their stuff on magazine covers, billboards, and television shows. We stare at them as we stand in line at the grocery store, as we drive down the highways, and as we gaze blankly at the TV screen. We can't escape them. Every time we stare, our shoulders slump, our bellies feel soft, and we grow a little more disappointed, thinking that fitness is something that's beyond our reach.

What a mess.

During the past 20 years, as the image of the ultimate fit body has become more and more impossible to obtain, we've become pudgier and pudgier. Every year, fewer and fewer people exercise. No matter how often we try to recharge our fitness pursuits, we seem to almost always fall off the wagon.

The latest *U.S. Surgeon General's Report on Physical Activity and Health* states that only 20 percent of Americans—that's 2 out of 10—exercise consistently three or four times a week, for one hour per session, at their target heart rates. Yet, we're bombarded with more than 7,000 health and fitness messages every year. Why don't we do what we know is good for us?

Because we haven't tapped into our fitness instincts.

HOW I DISCOVERED THE FITNESS INSTINCT

I've always been interested in fitness. After I graduated from college with a journalism degree, I tried to write stories about it, but I discovered that I didn't know what I was talking about. So I went back to school, got a nursing degree, became a cardiac care specialist, and founded the Aerobics and Fitness Association of America's *American Fitness* magazine.

I've been doing a lot of lectures since then. Nearly a decade ago, though, my entire outlook about fitness changed. I was talking to an audience of tremendously fit people, and I realized that most of my words were only going to make the fit fitter. I grew curious and frustrated about what the fitness industry calls the great unmotivated masses, the 80 percent of the population who are routinely described by the media as exercise and diet recalcitrants.

Thus, I started rounding up these "recalcitrants" and began asking them question after question. For three years, I conducted a national research project. I interviewed more than 400 formerly sedentary people from every walk of life who had successfully adopted healthy lifestyles. I asked them about their motivations to be fit and healthy. I charted the course of weary consumers who had labored under dashed hopes, pursuing impossible physiques and deceptive techniques, but who then discovered how to throw an inner switch that fueled their passions for the fit life—naturally!

During this time, I also traveled most of the world, studying the religions, philosophies, and fitness styles of ancient cultures. I immersed myself in the world of alternative medicine.

It took years of interviews, travel, and research for me to come to an amazingly simple realization: Each and every human being has within them an instinctive knowledge for optimal movement. Putting all my learnings together, I developed a simple, step-by-step, no-fail method for tapping into your fitness instinct, a revolutionary approach to holistic fitness. After you read *The Fitness Instinct*, exercise and play will become completely natural parts of your every waking hour. You'll find out how to tap into your seventh sense—your natural instinct for movement—which, once awakened, will guide your every stretch, run, jump, dance, pushup, and crunch. This book will give you life-enhancing findings that you can select and develop into your own tailor-made fitness program.

The Fitness Instinct is a first-time compilation of astounding new research from the West coupled with modern-day insights into the oldest disciplines of the East: yoga, tai chi, and qigong. In addition, the book explains how to incorporate into your life the secrets of the remarkably strong, flexible, and lean indigenous people of Nepal, Thailand, Peru, and the Sudan. In short, you will learn the Tao of Instinctive Movement, a blend of East and West.

I wrote *The Fitness Instinct* as the first fitness book for "the rest of us." Based on my extensive research, it offers the first real hope for you if you have ever:

- Been frustrated by your lack of commitment to an exercise program.
- Turned on your heels and headed out of health clubs, embarrassed and intimidated by the hard-bodies on full display.
- Had it with expensive equipment, unrealistic methods, and bogus promises.
- Hauled your stepper, stationary cycle, and rower to the garage, only to flush with shame every time you see the equipment covered with cobwebs.

LIBERATION FROM THE GYM

By reading this book, you will discover how to finally liberate yourself from the one-size-fits-all exercise prescription and the need for high-priced clubs and gimmicks. You'll learn a valuable new strategy that abandons such sacred cows as conventional routines that require ironclad discipline, repetitive drudgery, logs, and diaries.

By following the 11-step method described in these pages, you will be able to enjoy an approach to fitness that is whole, healthy, and in harmony with your life. You'll effortlessly leap over your past hurdles to fitness. You'll actually begin to love movement. You'll never dread another workout.

Really. I'm not kidding.

You see, the whole problem with fitness—the real reason that you don't exercise as much as you want to—centers on being out of touch with your body. Too many of us force ourselves through boring routines that make us feel like automatons.

There are sound reasons that much of the fitness movement has failed to turn you on. Fitness itself, with all of its exercise prescriptions and training recommendations, is dry, boring, and out of touch with your personal interests, psychology, and emotions. Fitness trainers and exercise experts have made fitness harder than it really is, thus robbing you of your own intuitive know-how.

It's no wonder that we skip our exercise plans when something—any-thing—comes up. It's not that we're not motivated. It's simply that we haven't found moves that we enjoy.

Until now.

I've traveled the world and attended just about every fitness class imagin-able, and I've discovered plenty of moves that aren't boring. In fact, they're fun. They're moves that you can actually look forward to. I've described them all in this book.

You'll also learn how to tap into your natural instinct to move—your sev-enth sense—as well as your natural storehouse of inspiration, intuition, and motivation.

A BETTER PATH

Yes, there's a much better way. Take this new finding: An 80-year-old or-chestra conductor doing nothing more than waving his arms in front of the musicians can experience a greater surge of endorphins than a tightly wound, overworked, and overstressed corporate executive pounding out his Stair-master workout and throwing perspiration like a lawn sprinkler. How can this be? Enjoyment. The mind-body factor. Researchers in the new field of psy-choneuroimmunology (how our thoughts affect our bodies) always suspected that it was powerful, but they are just now beginning to realize to what extent.

Research shows that persisting with exercises that you find boring or re-gard as acts of mind over matter will eventually backfire. There is a disqui-eting, dispiriting effect that occurs when you consistently coerce your body to perform odious actions. After "being good" for a while, you succumb to a veg-etative stupor for days. If you're like most people, I bet that you've experi-enced this backfire before. It's a response that's similar to the well-cited deprivation-binge cycle noted by dieting experts.

Sometimes, a more harmful response occurs: You get sick. Chronic fatigue syndrome, autoimmune diseases, allergies, and certain cancers affect the over-achieving exercise crowd. On the other hand, heart disease, high blood pres-sure, diabetes, and obesity plague the sedentary. Both ends of the fit-unfit continuum reflect poor health. How do we strike a balance?

With holistic fitness.

Instead of prescribing the same formula in a sea of sound-alike, look-alike fitness books, holistic fitness appears like a blast of fresh air in an overcrowded sweat shop. Holistic fitness contains the missing links that allow everybody— from neophytes to exercise dropouts—to finally jump on the endorphin bandwagon. What's more, the holistic fitness approach in *The Fitness Instinct* gives a motivation boost even to hard-core fitness fanatics who've grown staid and uninspired in their routines. I've included advice on diversifying and spicing up your routine if you've already discovered the joys of fitness but are seeking some fresh ideas.

THE 11-STEP PLAN

The Fitness Instinct puts the "fit" back in fitness, and the timing couldn't be better. An exciting array of new research has begun poking holes in the outworn bastion of what's conventionally preached as "the right way to exercise." As I've said, this book contains illuminating research, never before presented.

You see, the reason that you don't exercise has nothing to do with your willpower or natural ability. Rather, it has to do with a fitness industry that seems bent on squashing your body's own natural know-how. You'll learn more about that in chapter 1.

Then I'll take you on a fascinating 11-step journey, a blueprint that will eliminate the most common barriers to adopting lasting health and fitness habits and regaining your natural impulses for self-care. I discovered from my research and experience that this can be accomplished through the following steps.

Get to know yourself. You can't tap into your inner wisdom until you know who you are. The self-tests in chapter 2 will help you uncover hidden traits that make you most suited for particular types of movement. Remember your movement personality. It will pop up over and over again throughout the book.

Learn the truth. Unrealistic expectations may be the biggest barrier to adopting lasting health habits. Not doing enough. Not achieving *that* body. Distorted perceptions fostered by celebrity-obsessed media and the fitness industry run women and men ragged, chipping away at self-esteem and throwing up monstrous obstacles to integrating a healthy lifestyle. Yet, people told me that the minute they decided to unhook from the fitness industry "scene," they regained their sense of what was good for them.

With knowledge of your fitness personality firmly in hand, chapter 3 will help you confront and let go of these previously unquestioned assumptions about achieving fitness. The 15 lies—heavily promoted by the fitness industry—that I expose in this chapter stand in the way of instinctual fitness. (*Warning*: Some of these lies may anger and shock you.)

Believe in yourself. Many of us pick up destructive beliefs and thoughts throughout our lives. For instance, if you think, "I'll probably never be fit. I've just never been any good at it," or "The best way to motivate myself is by posting my sky-high cholesterol results by the treadmill," you have some issues to confront. Chapter 4 will help you do that. You see, negative thinking—in any shape or form—will squash your natural body wisdom, keeping you from doing what's best for your body. This chapter outlines the top seven self-sabotaging thoughts and the five best ways to get them out of your head.

Relax, rest, and rejuvenate. If you've ever forced yourself to exercise—dragged yourself to an aerobics class even though you didn't want to be there—you know all too well that you can't force yourself to exercise for very long.

Here's a better way: Don't. Instead, exercise in a mindful, centered, restful place. To do so, you must first destress, relax, and find your still point, the place where all mindful movement starts. Chapter 5 will teach you 15 different ways to find this contemplative state that allows you to make any permanent change that is needed.

Listen to your body. It's talking to you. Your seventh sense is your natural instinct for movement. Suppress it, and you shrivel up. Awaken it, and you have a life partner for good health.

Your seventh sense is coaxing you to move. To hear it talking to you, follow my four steps in chapter 6. Here, you'll learn how to scan your body to determine when and how it wants to move. This body check will replace the drudgery of exercise with your idea of a welcome, joyful movement experience.

Let time move you. Are you a morning person, bounding out of bed full of energy and life? Or are you a night owl, staying up late, ready to rock and roll at 10:00 P.M.? It makes a difference. Because of circadian rhythms, your body responds differently to movement at different times of the day. This is a natural process, but many times we ignore it and try to power through it. To paraphrase the song, there's a time for rest, a time for energizing moves, a time for stretching, and a time for strengthening. Chapter 7 will teach you which moves work best for you at which times of day. You'll learn how to feel and respond to the urging of time, treating yourself to a grand movement excursion right at the peak of your energy cycle.

Move with flow. When you find flow, you know it. Suddenly, you're totally absorbed in what you're doing. You lose track of time. You don't hear the phone ring. In fact, you can even forget to eat! You enjoy what you are doing and how you are feeling, and you wish it could last forever.

Imagine feeling this way about exercise. Chapter 8 provides 19 different ways to tap into such flow states while you're moving. These moves lower stress, optimize pleasure, and are right in step with your seventh sense.

Move in spurts. When I did a time analysis of various people's daily routines of work, home life, family responsibilities, and errands, I realized that these people were actually already performing a significant amount of energy output, and they didn't even know it. A working mom, for instance, would charge around from 6:00 A.M. to 10:00 P.M., surpassing the calorie expenditure recommended on most charts for daily exercise. Her time spent in sedentary pursuits, such as sitting in front of the TV in the evenings, was not unreasonable when taken as part of her overall 24-hour action-rest cycle.

Too many of us have failed at traditional fitness routines because we believed what the fitness industry told us: We had to "work out" for an hour at least three or four times a week. You don't. In fact, you shouldn't.

Your body wasn't designed to move hard for only a few hours a week. It's simply not natural. Nor was it made to sit still for hours. Chapter 9 will teach you how to move in spurts all day long, burning more calories and building more fitness than you would with the older, traditional methods. It's a better, more natural, more intuitive way to move.

Find hidden inspiration. Many people make the mistake of hiring personal trainers to motivate them to exercise. That's okay to learn new techniques, but to motivate yourself, you can simply reclaim your "inner trainer." (You'll learn how in chapter 10.) Your natural inspiration and intuition can guide your every move. You'll find both in some surprising places: dreams, deep breaths, spiritual teachings, sunsets, and even family gatherings.

Overflow with motivation. We sometimes force ourselves into exercise, believing that we're suffering from a lack of motivation. We're just not tapping fully into our natural storehouse of motivation. In chapter 11, you'll find out how to use rewards, goals, and mindfulness to spur yourself into action. Best yet, you'll tap into your core desire, a genuine passion that can make you accomplish just about any task, including fitness. Once you learn your core desire, no task will seem insurmountable.

Stay realistic. Deep down, most of us are tempted by quick fixes for self-enhancement. Society places enormous pressure on us to look, act, and feel thin, young, and sexy. Thus, no matter how much we learn to accept ourselves the way we are, deep down, we usually still wish for a quick fix. The diet that will really lop off 10 pounds. The body cream that will really make cellulite disappear. Chapter 12 shows you how to deal with such wishful thinking as well as which quick fixes actually might be worth your time.

GET READY TO THROW THE SWITCH

With *The Fitness Instinct*, you will bypass all of the old excuses for not exercising. You're about to learn and enjoy guilt-free, pleasurable techniques that are simple, direct, lifesaving, accessible, and either free or affordable.

The good news is finally here. Embracing the fit life is not a matter of willpower or genetic luck. If you perform the simple self-assessments and practice the daily steps described here, you will build confidence as you look better, feel healthier, and enjoy life more fully. *The Fitness Instinct* truly is a revolutionary approach to fitness. It is my sincere hope that you have fun with these techniques, learn to play more with the liberating spirit of movement in your life, and thoroughly enjoy the rewards of holistic fitness.

When it's all said and done, what makes some people never lift themselves off the couch while others take good care of themselves? Again, dozens of reasons emerge—financial hardship, geographic inconvenience, time constraints, overwhelming family demands—but basically, I've found that, plain and simple, they have not thrown the switch yet.

What will you find in this book that's going to make you take good care of yourself? You will learn to activate an internal switch—the energizing charge that keeps you at the center of your decision-making switchboard. You're about to embody an internal authority and body sovereignty and experience fitness from the inside out, rather than following externally imposed dictates.

You're about to embrace your birthright of daily, enjoyable movement. Human life insists on movement at every stage: Chromosomes square dance to form a new being, and the dying breath shakes its farewell rattle. When movement is natural and intrinsically driven, mind, body, and spirit come into harmony. The internal impulse to move and stretch and dance and walk is one grand caress. When women and men awaken to the miracle of life dancing within them, the motivation to be fit, with all of its culturally ingrained judgments, obsessions, and beliefs, recedes from the shores like the last frantic wave at the end of a storm. Left in the glittering sun is the celebration of life. Embracing yourself, you move once again for the pure joy of it.

Let's begin.

chapter 1

Why the Fitness Bandwagon Has Passed By So Many

It's time to compare the promise to the reality. For 25 years, the fitness cartel has spent millions of dollars convincing us that the pursuit of hard bodies is the key to happiness. This relentless message has persuaded a few to become full-time fanatics, while the vast majority of us have fallen by the wayside, watching as the fitness bandwagon rolls by. Perhaps you are one of that majority.

Don't feel guilty. It's not your fault if you don't exercise. It's not your fault if your body doesn't look like Jane Fonda's or Arnold Schwarzenegger's. It's not your fault if the thought of pumping iron, wearing revealing spandex, jumping to an aerobics instructor's bark, and generally breathing hard and breaking a sweat makes you want to hide under your bed.

Blame it on the fitness industry.

Much of the reason that you may hate exercise can be attributed to the way fitness has been sold and packaged. A split in the population has occurred between the 20 percent who have benefited from the fitness industry's message and the 80 percent who have been left behind, frustrated and gaining more weight every year. This 20/80 split continues despite a lot of lip service at many health clubs about just going for good health and forgetting about perfection. No matter what is said by the staffs and personal trainers, the emphasis, messages, and images speak louder than the latest politically correct spin.

Two out of 10 people find that the hard-body, muscle-mania approach at health clubs is just their ticket. Still, not even those in this minority reap the full benefits of movement. Even these successfully serious exercisers report—both in scientific studies and in my own research—that their fitness pursuits fail to awaken deep, abiding feelings of self-worth and well-being. Rather, their fitness quests often fuel their obsessions about shortcomings and make them feel worse about themselves, their efforts, and their bodies.

As for the other 80 percent, they fall prey to something that I call the intimidation factor, that dreadful sense of shrinking inward and wanting to disappear that you feel when you enter unsafe territory. More than two-thirds of the people I've interviewed talked about the distress they felt when surrounded by "perfect bodies." Diane, a 28-year-old former gymnast, told me that she felt "awkward and incompetent" around the weight equipment, "as if everyone is staring at me, knowing I'm not using much resistance." An older computer engineer told me that he was so embarrassed about his out-of-shape body that he left the gym within a few minutes, without finishing his routine. "The trainers and regulars already have their little clique going. They can't help but hang around and laugh together. I knew that I was the source of their amusement, so I got the heck out. You won't find me exercising around perfect bodies ever again."

Whether that perfection was real or imagined is another story. I honestly believe that there is no "perfect body." None of the people I talked to—not even those who had what almost any of us would call perfect bodies—considered themselves to be without imperfections. Even cover models groaned about their skinny calves or their puny wrists or their low-set ears, as if the Earth's rotation depended on their having a different appearance. Why? The pursuit of perfection has been drummed into us with a million images, launching a million obsessions.

Starting at a very early age, girls and boys tend to adopt dieting habits and anxieties about body image based on seductive ads and images designed to sell the perfect body. For years, we all watched Kellogg's Special K commercials in which a slinky torso, the headless woman of a million ads, glided around in a swimsuit. In 1998, however, Kellogg's decided to challenge the stereotypes that have fueled women's insecurities. The cereal-maker began creating ads that debunk the ideal body image, announcing that "perfection is about accepting yourself the way you are," says Karen Kafer, the firm's director of communications. A more recent ad features a worried-looking, naked baby girl with a caption balloon: "Do I look fat?"

Self-esteem is largely determined by how people feel about their looks. I didn't want to believe this, and I hoped that self-esteem was determined more by one's education, social support, family ties, and similar high-minded standards. Then I reviewed more than 300 research studies and psychological surveys that convinced me otherwise. At the same time, as a television journalist, I was regularly coached by media consultants who showed me the focus group statistics about what people remember.

When people listen to a speaker, the visual content accounts for 70 percent of what they recall. They pay attention to only about 10 percent of the words. That's why, when Hillary and Bill Clinton went on prime-time TV during the 1992 campaign to talk about surmounting marriage difficulties, all people could talk about the next day was Hillary's hairdo. We're just a little strange that way. Disconcerting as this was, I saw how the fitness industry could easily prey upon this natural tendency to focus on the image and, in turn, let the image affect our feelings of self-worth.

WHAT IS FITNESS, ANYWAY?

Let's be clear about this. Fitness isn't anything real or tangible. You can't go out and buy some "fitness." Nor can you store it, save it for a rainy day, or share it. Some people think that they never have enough of it, although others would look at them and believe that fitness is the main thing they have going for them. Fitness is a concept, a word, an image in the mind, shaped by decades of advances in exercise science along with corporate-sponsored images and publicly broadcast messages. Fitness as a cultural phenomenon is controlled by a cartel that includes several industries, among them beauty, fashion, sports, sporting goods, and media. What is *real* is your life.

It's easy to lose sight of that when fitness is packaged and sold in the image of a mean-looking tigress wearing a very revealing leotard to show off a bosom that defies nature—not to mention gravity—on someone with such obviously low body fat. Just in case the message is too subtle for you, the tigress is usually posed in profile, with her spine dramatically arched and her butt thrust out. This pose has launched many million-dollar aerobics video careers and sold millions of dollars worth of health club memberships, fitness equipment, clothing, and beauty products.

This unrealistic and unattainable image can turn you into a mere spectator in life. When you can shake off the spectator trance, however, and return to your own life, you get to explore what fitness can mean specifically for you. In other words, what matters to you physically is your ability to perform all of the activities of a typical day. Now, if your typical day involves a lot of back arching and butt thrusting, perhaps the fitness cartel can help you. If not, it's time to help yourself.

If you had to run down your food, chasing rabbits and guinea pigs as do the people of a native tribe in northern Mexico, fitness would imply the ability to sprint like a cheetah every other day. If you earned your daily keep by diving for sponges, you would be fit only if you could hold your breath for three minutes. Keeping up a level of fitness that exceeds your present daily activity requires an artificial overlay of exercise. By artificial, I mean any physical effort that is not part of your normal movement repertoire.

We go through the days performing about four or five different movements: stretching, lifting, reaching, walking, and holding. These moves help us to be functionally fit to accomplish what we want. They exercise the entire neuromuscular unit, from brain to limbs and back again. Think of it as a loop of fired-up electrons, a lightning stream of neurons and twitchy muscles,

---

REAL FITNESS I asked different types of people what their ideas of exercise were. Not some celebrity's or fitness trainer's definition or some advice from a column, but their own ideas. Here's what they told me.

- "Playing in the dirt," said a 76-year-old grandmother who loved to garden.
- "Dancing like there's no tomorrow," laughed a Hispanic couple who dig ballroom dancing but never build it into their weekly schedule.
- "Acting like a kid," said a young father who only has time to roughhouse with his brawny toddler.
- "Mall jammin'" confirmed a group of seventh graders with a penchant for retail aerobics.
- "Shreddin' till you're hollow," insisted two snowboarders who were obviously ready for lunch.
- "Taking a tumble," offered instructors at the Broadway Gymnastics club.
- "Gliding on the water," said a rowing team in Boston Harbor.

communicating and cooperating. As wellness expert Neil Sol, Ph.D., explains, "Functional fitness is all about strengthening the loop." If that's the case, artificial exercise ignores the loop.

Isolating one muscle with a slow set of carefully tracked bicep curls is, in a sense, an artificial exercise. Rarely in life do you have to use one muscle to do something. The act of reaching for a heavy dictionary and lifting it across a table involves numerous muscles in your shoulders, chest, and arms—more muscles and tendons than you can imagine. Some work as primary movers, others as secondary assistants, and still others as stabilizers. An entire concert of cooperative teamwork takes place.

Time spent performing isolated movements and artificial exercise is part of the cult of body image and perfection obsession. The more hours you invest in this cult, the more you invest in the world of image over substance, looks over function. How did this happen? It happened because fitness became mystified.

THE MYSTIFICATION OF FITNESS

Making it harder than it is—that's how any profession robs you of your own intuitive know-how. The legal profession invented its own legalese. The medical profession created an aura of "knowing better" about life-and-death issues. Even mortgage institutions know how to make a homeowner's agreement so convoluted that you willingly pay all sorts of fees just to free yourself from the excruciating explanation of details.

The fitness profession is no different. Health and fitness have become mystified, abstracted, and intellectualized. We now must rely on scientists and experts, instead of our own common sense, to figure out how to be fit. I've been asked by countless people, "What should I do if I don't like going to a gym or working with weights?"—as if simple movements such as walking or dancing were somehow beyond their normal experience. They ask, "What kind of exercise should I do if I've got the flu?"—as if they have lost their bodily cues to lie down, rest, and recover. I grow more dismayed every day when I read letters to the editor asking, "Is walking really a good way to exercise?"—as if the simple act and its blood-pumping benefits elude them. Inquirers ask about intensity, "How do I know if I'm working too hard?"—as if they can't tell anymore when their muscles are tired or they are out of breath.

Of course, people believe that they need these answers in order to exercise properly. If you've listened to the countless messages dumped on your doorstep by the fitness industry, you've probably believed it, too—until now. You shouldn't feel like a dope for relying on these fitness "experts" for answers that your body already knows. You've been brainwashed—and now it's time to undo the damage.

Many people have lost touch with their own bodies' yearnings to stretch, move, walk, or dance. Ever since the new breed of experts largely requisitioned fitness training and physical advice, I have discovered in more than 400 interviews how a reasonable person's own self-generating capacity for initiating movement is polluted with embarrassment and insecurity.

The fitness industry has simply made health and fitness information difficult to understand. Mystification takes fitness out of the practical and into the scientific realm, requiring high levels of mastery. Exercise science mastery became the exclusive domain of specialists who had achieved advanced levels of education and experience: sports medicine physicians, exercise physiologists, cardiac nurse specialists, certified technicians—professionals who must interpret the scientific data and write your exercise prescription. This orientation was borrowed from the development of cardiac rehabilitation programs, which blossomed in the 1980s due to the record number of coronary bypass operations.

Government public health officials, together with the American Heart Association (AHA) and cardiac researchers, started identifying the risk factors linked to heart disease. In a scramble to control or lower those risk factors, entire protocols were developed to help people change their behavior. As new findings developed, we altered the programs, but for decades, they stayed fairly consistent in recommending the following strategies.

- Limit dietary fat to no more than 30 percent of total calories.
- Lower cholesterol below 200 milligrams and triglycerides under 120.
- Don't smoke.
- Control blood pressure by keeping the systolic reading below 140 and the diastolic number below 90.
- Practice some form of stress management.
- Maintain your ideal weight.
- Perform consistent aerobic exercise.

For years, highly publicized national campaigns shouted that if people would only follow these recommendations, they could beat the odds and lower their risks of heart attacks and strokes. It was only when we had many individuals who were still having heart attacks despite doing everything we recommended that we began to question what other biological, emotional, psychological, and genetic factors might be at work.

When I was a cardiac care nurse, for example, I knew a 40-year-old runner who surpassed every one of those guidelines. He followed a heart-healthy diet, even sprinkling lecithin (a fat emulsifier) on his breakfast cereal. He had the blood pressure of a teenager. He had no family history of heart disease or any other identifiable risk factors. Thus, when he dropped dead from a sudden heart attack, it made me question the value of the numbers game. How do we continue to counsel people to follow set-in-stone guidelines, when every day we see men and women who don't fit the risk factor description yet still succumb to the chief killer of our time?

What the young runner had working against him was the heartbreak of a recent divorce. At that time, grief and loneliness were not part of the scientific profile for heart disease. More recently, however, the case for emotional pain and isolation as risk factors has begun to make its way into the medical literature. It seems that heartbreak is linked to heart disease, and loneliness impacts the immune system.

After working in cardiac care units, I became the cardiac rehabilitation supervisor at a major heart center in Los Angeles; at the same time, I was starting *American Fitness* magazine and writing videos and texts for fitness instructors. It seemed like a perfect segue, since cardiac rehabilitation principles were emulated in the fitness field. Every lifestyle lesson taught to the at-risk population was now being preached to everyone else—now ominously referred to as the "apparently healthy" population. The word *apparently* changed the entire timbre of the fitness movement, allowing nonmedical fitness personnel, armed with the oft-quoted quasi-statistic that "1 in 4 Americans is at risk for heart attack or stroke," to cast a suspicious eye on the average man or woman. (The actual rate is 1 in 1,000, but "at risk" can encompass any number of factors, including stress or physical inactivity.) This misleading statement was latched on to by the health club owners as an advertising ploy, while their staffs scrambled for CPR certification.

THE LAND OF WALKING TIME BOMBS

Clients were seen as "walking time bombs," reported one fitness center employee. "We were scared that they would drop dead of heart attacks during their warmups." Club enrollments included medical disclaimers as well as the usual lawsuit waivers; many clubs followed through with extensive client self-reports outlining medical histories and cardiac risk profiles.

In all fairness, some clients really were at risk for cardiac trouble. For example, I was called as an expert witness to testify against a health club that failed to ask the appropriate questions of a 28-year-old, overweight African-American man who had high blood pressure. After complaining to the staff that he didn't feel well, he was encouraged to take another few runs around the track before going to the steam room. There, he collapsed from a major heart attack and was finally rushed to an emergency room. His rocky hospitalization left him on disability for life.

In their depositions, the club owners talked about the "out-of-shape, unfit characters" and "lazy, unmotivated lard-butts" who "didn't have the proper drive to get fit." I was appalled by their insensitive and self-righteous attitudes, but I knew that the tide had turned against them as far as negligence litigation was concerned. The health club chain settled out of court for an undisclosed sum.

I think about this man now and wonder what could have saved him from a life of baby-sitting his black-and-blue heart. Just how far did he get from knowing what was physically good for him and what wasn't? When he was goaded into taking those treacherous jogs around the track, all the while feeling a crushing pain in his left shoulder and nausea rising in his throat, didn't he stop and think, "This isn't such a good idea; my body can't take this right now"?

I had a chance to ask these questions. This former IBM junior manager is now in his late thirties, still on disability, divorced, and struggling with day-to-day physical exertion. He talked about the tremendous amount of intimidation he felt from the moment he entered the health club. "Everyone was really buff, really in shape. I told them that I had read in their ad in the paper that they had 'personal counselors' who could tailor-make a program for me. I knew I was out of shape. I hadn't done anything since high school, and I knew I had high blood pressure, but they didn't ask any questions. They just told me to go and stand with a group of ladies in leotards and somebody would show us the ropes. I asked them again about the personalized part, but they said that everybody got the same thing in the beginning." So much for individual counseling and tailored training.

He also told me that he reported his discomfort and nausea over and over but was told, "Look, that's just nerves. You're probably looking for an excuse to quit—everybody does in the beginning. Just push through it."

What bothers me most about this response is not the lack of exercise knowledge that obviously produced it but rather the mean-spirited discounting of an individual's genuine fears. I believe unconscionable reactions such as this reflect an arrogance and steel-edged superiority that are fostered by the strength-training and body-shaping cults of the fitness movement. Their script goes like this: "I know what's better for you than you do . . . so just pay up and shut up."

"IS IT OKAY TO BEND OVER?"

Some personal trainers consider themselves the priests of the fitness religion, serving as intermediaries between the handed-down commandments of body expertise (to which they alone have access) and you. As a whole, the profession has done a lot of good, but I've interviewed far too many health-club members to not make this critique. Often, the trainers have the last word not only about your protocol and progress but also about what constitutes peak performance for you. In interview after interview, I heard women and men complain that they are "so out of shape" that they need personal trainers to harass them into exercise regimens they hate but believe they should do anyway.

At this point, the fitness cartel has usurped basic body knowledge to the extent that the average person I interviewed believes that she can no longer trust her sensory awareness. "The advice keeps changing every year. I've lost my instinct to know what's good for me," complained Shelly, a mother of two who has been a chronic dieter and sometime gym-goer for more than 15 years. She talked about how she tried to follow exercise classes that promised weight loss but steadily gained 15 pounds a year for quite a while. One year's advice was that fat burning is accomplished through low-intensity, long-duration exercise. Another year's advice was that it is accomplished through overall calorie burn, no matter what the intensity.

People write to health and fitness columnists in newspapers nationwide with questions such as: "What do I do to lose weight?" "How long should I walk?" "Should I jump rope?" "Will dumbbells hurt my back?" As unbelievable as it may seem, I got a flurry of questions regarding the simple act of

REAL-LIFE INSTINCTS

After Vickie injured her hip, she joined a health club with a pool. She looked forward to walking in the warm water. She knew that the gentle resistance of the water could help her regain her strength after being unable to do much of anything for several weeks. However, the personal trainers at the gym stood in her way. "I have faced discrimination all my life, since I got fat at the age of five," she says. "From the moment I walked in for my fitness assessment, I knew I was in trouble."

The average weight of the five women and one man in the fitness assessment area was about 130 pounds. None of them looked more than 25 years old. Nobody could understand Vickie's challenges. "I am 44 and fat. I know that. It's not a big mystery. I was passed from one to the other like a sack of potatoes so they could do their tests on me," she says. "I was humiliated. Worst of all, the one man in the group was the one to take my measurements and use the calipers to do my body-fat analysis. His expression was grim. He told me that he would have to inactivate my access card until a doctor had a chance to evaluate my information and decide whether I was a risk. It didn't matter to them that I had already been using the pool for a week with no ill effects. I couldn't do it anymore. I wasn't acceptable."

Unfortunately, there are millions of Vickies out there. Maybe you know one, or maybe you are one. The real tragedy is that Vickie instinctively knew that walking in the pool was the ideal healing movement for her. She wasn't asking to jog around the track or lift a stack of weights. She understood that gentle exercise was called for. She was her own trainer, not the so-called experts at the gym.

bending over to tie one's shoes. This quandary was prompted after a leading fitness organization banned "prolonged unsupported forward flexion."

Often, I've been asked to ghost-write question-and-answer columns for celebrities such as Arnold Schwarzenegger and many others. "Supply people with brief and helpful answers to all their questions," was the innocent-sounding proposal. I've done these columns for years in national publications, and the questions seem to grow more and more out of touch. A growing dependency develops whenever I supply people with answers to questions that are best asked of themselves. There is only one response to all of these questions that has integrity: Return the question in an empowering way and help people develop awareness about their own body responses.

That's what I hope to do for you with this book—help you answer your own fitness questions. For instance, here's a sampling of common questions to which you already know the answers.

What do I do to lose weight? Ask yourself, "What has worked for me in the past?"

How long should I walk? Ask yourself, "How long do I feel comfortable walking?"

Should I jump rope? Ask yourself, "How do I feel when I try it?"

Will dumbbells hurt my back? Ask yourself, "Does my back hurt now? What aggravates it?"

Reflective questioning helps to establish that you—yes, you—are best-suited to determine how your body feels with movement. Anything short of that fosters dependency and robs you of basic self-knowledge about your body.

There are many well-intentioned professionals in the fitness industry who recognize that the old paradigm isn't working and who are asking for a new approach. I'm on the road quite a bit, delivering speeches, workshops, and keynote presentations to people in the health, wellness, and fitness fields. I'm often asked what I recommend for health and fitness promoters, and I tell them that it starts with the basics: Learn to listen and ask questions first. Just as doctors and pharmacists are learning to drop their arrogance and stubbornness and finally listen to patients, it's important for fitness promoters—who are, in essence, part of an offshoot of the medical profession—to follow suit. I tell them to start any counseling session not with their own agendas and well-rehearsed prescriptions in mind but with a sincere attempt to understand the client's life and goals.

Second, I tell health-care providers that they have to finally understand that the population has split into two groups: the 20 percent who are disciplined in their fitness routines, and the 80 percent who are turned off by it all. I tell them that if health and fitness professionals really want to make a difference, they have to listen to the stories of the 80 percent. It was only by listening closely to those tales that I learned to set aside my own arrogance and judgments as a health professional. I also had to come to terms with the ways that I had helped create and colluded with an industry that reinforced messages and images that were, on second look, at cross-purposes to the happiness and goals of 8 out of 10 people. In fact, much of the fitness message that I and others were spreading was antagonistic. By dropping what I thought I knew and listening deeply, I started my own journey of self-healing and transformation as well.

Four years of interviewing brought me to my knees professionally, and I knew that I couldn't go on doing what I had been doing. The interviews revealed an unbridgeable gap between the oft-hailed "health habits" that people are supposed to follow and what they are actually able to accomplish each day; between the motivational techniques that we encourage people to employ and the irritating discontent and unhappiness that these techniques leave in their wake. With interview after interview and story after story, I learned and awakened and publicly asked for forgiveness. This book is a collection of what I learned and what I saw that truly does work for those who are able to break away from the fitness cartel's grasp and learn once again to listen to—and trust—their own bodies.

ARE YOU WORTH THE EFFORT?

In almost every interview that I conducted, it came down to the same thing. As people started to roll out their long, sad list of excuses for why they didn't exercise or eat right, they often ended with a shrug of the shoulders, declaring, "It's not worth the effort." Upon further questioning, that statement started to unfold into "*I'm* not worth the effort." Similarly, another discounting phrase, "I didn't try hard enough," often turned into "I'm not good enough." For some it was, "I don't have what it takes." Countless women repeated a similar version: "I don't know what's wrong with me—I just can't stick to the diet and exercise routine they taught me."

What do we have here? An epidemic of low self-esteem? A contagion of self-deprecating remarks permeates the fitness attitude of the average person. I asked many leading health promotion experts what could contribute to this malaise. Nationally renowned professionals such as Pat Lyons, R.N., a leading educator at Kaiser Permanente Health System in California, founder of Connections, Women's Health Consulting Network, and co-author of *Great Shape*; Steve Ramirez, head of the Fresno County health services in California; and Michael O'Donnell, Ph.D., editor of the *American Journal of Health Promotion*, all agree: The experts have been proselytizing people with the same message for more than 20 years and watching them fail at consistent change. This sets up a cycle of blame and repeat failure that sends people into downward spirals of gaining more weight and becoming more sedentary. One wellness physician at the Veteran Administrations Hospital in Los Angeles described this cycle in this way.

> *It's gotten so that I don't tell anybody what to do anymore—and that's a huge shift for a doctor, believe me. Instead of assigning this ridiculously artificial routine on a Health Rider or some other piece of equipment that they hate and that is going to be thrown in the garage in a week, I just listen to them about how they conduct their days—where they work, what they like to do when they come home. I'm beginning to think that it all comes down to self-esteem. If they start to feel good about themselves, I can assist that process by showing some interest in them as people instead of seeing them as people who need to alter their entire lifestyles. And that's another thing: Alter for whom? For them, or for me, so I feel better about my medical practice? They've got to make the change from within, and I'm convinced that it actually starts with self-esteem.*

THE HIGH-PRICED RIP-OFF

To understand how insane the fitness movement has become, consider the case of Gayle, the single mother of a six-year-old boy, who works two jobs just to make ends meet. She has always carried 10 more pounds than she'd like, and late one night, she succumbed to the propaganda of an infomercial selling a $150 walking program. By the time we talked, the question she had begun to ask herself was, "Do I really need a $150 program, complete with audiocassettes, training heart zones, walking exercise zones, motivational tapes, and life-size posters of walking celebrities—*in order to take a walk?*"

Here is her description of the expensive walking program, endorsed by a fitness celebrity, that she purchased from TV.

> *I was disappointed the minute I got it—not so much in the package but in myself for falling for another gimmick. I mean, look at my day: I run around like a chicken with her head cut off all day, in and out of errands, chasing around like crazy. Then, I finally get home from work, change my clothes, throw some dinner in the oven for my son, Joey, and strap on the headphones to listen to my audio walking program. I figure*

I can take a quick walk around the block at least. It's been a week since I bought this thing; I'd better use it.

I don't have time to read the booklet, which looks like it basically says something about three walking speeds: slow, medium, and fast. Hello?! This is unbelievable. What did I pay for this? I don't want to think about it.

Anyway, I can't stand it. I want to get going, but the tape is blabbing about all the safety factors and risks of walking—stuff I should know before I get started. I've wasted about 10 minutes on my front porch and haven't moved a step. Maybe I have the wrong tape. I go back in the house to see if there's at least some music I can listen to, and then I want to break down and cry. What am I doing? Did I really need this to go take a walk?

No, Gayle did not need to go through this aggravation and expense in order to take a walk. Somewhere along the line, though, she came to believe that other people know better about what is good for her, so she transferred authority outside herself and looked to the experts for answers about something as basic as taking a walk. When we arrived at this insight in her interview, she got teary-eyed and shook her head, saying, "I'm really done with that routine."

Then, as if the universe were serving up a synchronous challenge, the phone rang in her home. Gayle talked a few minutes, asked some questions hesitantly, then wrote down an appointment. She hung up the phone and said, "That was the dentist's office. They said that I need another cleaning, even though I just had one a couple of months ago. But they said I needed one anyway, so I've got an appointment for that. I just hate the way they poke at the gum . . ." She stopped talking, maybe because of the look on my face; then she said, with a shocked look, "Oh, my God, I'm doing it again, aren't I?"

The conditioning is tougher to break than most people realize, but you must break this pattern in order to fully tap into your fitness instinct. In this book, I'll show you how to become aware of the very moment that your mind starts drifting into this dangerous territory and how to put a stop to it. Better yet, I'll show you how to come up with your own, more enlightened answers to whatever fitness question pops into your brain.

I am not saying that you should never ask anyone for help. Obviously,

REINSPIRING THE CHILDREN

With the wide variety of low-fat and nonfat food that is available today, why are teens fatter than ever? It's because they're sitting on the couch, watching TV and playing computer games. They're not exercising.

Lack of physical activity is an epidemic among kids. While parents may be able to influence the behavior of young school-age children by enrolling them in soccer and taking them on family outings, for the most part, kids drop out of physical exercise as they move into the teenage years. Over the past decade, the fitness participation of 12- to 17-year-olds has dropped 21 percent. Fewer than one in four children gets 30 minutes of any type of activity—moderate or vigorous—every day.

Next to the abundant and noisy marketing of fatty foods, the second biggest factor in teenage obesity is this sad decline in physical activity that occurs during adolescence. Believe it or not, only one state still mandates daily physical education classes at the high school level; in the other 49, participation has become optional. It's no surprise, then, that at the nation's high schools, enrollment in daily physical education classes dropped from 42 percent in 1991 to 25 percent in 1995.

The children are losing not only valuable lessons learned from sports, such as cooperation, but also the development of skills that give a boost to their self-images. A child who cannot play games will have a harder time staying fit.

What can you do about it? Be the best role model you can for young children and teens by enjoying a wide variety of active pastimes yourself. Cycle with them. Play games with them. Show them your commitment to daily physical activity. Involve them in sports and recreational activities. Become a volunteer coach. Insist that your school board hire physical education specialists, rather than just dumping this responsibility onto other teachers. Finally, limit children's TV viewing to no more than an hour a day.

You should also support the efforts of the chief organization that works to ensure that your children have abundant opportunities for healthy activities: the American Alliance for Health, Physical Education, Recreation, and Dance (AAHPERD). For more ideas, contact them at 1900 Association Drive, Reston, VA 20191.

when we are at a stage of initial learning or are not quite competent at a skill, depending on expert advice adds to our knowledge base. Usually, however, we already have the answers. We just need to learn to trust our bodies.

I did discover that women have a harder time with this than men. The cultural pressures on women to give up authority are unrelenting; the silencing act begins early. Psychologists Carol Gilligan, author of *In a Different Voice*, and Emily Hancock, author of *The Girl Within*, have both written about the stages in which young girls no longer assertively voice their opinions and even turn against their own instinctual natures. In a man's world, girls are expected to act coy, appear helpless, feel weaker, and show restraint. Not really saying what you think, coupled with constantly seeing images that are impossible to imitate but that the culture holds up as desirable, can erode your sense of self.

The inevitable next step seems to be, "If I'm not going to be in charge of what I think or feel, who will?" Tragically, there is an overabundance of tabloid cultural images to rush in to fill the vacuum. Young women not only silence what they think, they internalize what the culture says. I gave a talk to 25 young women, ages 16 to 18. I asked them which would be easier, to give me three full names of supermodels or tell me the date of their last period. They all opted for the supermodels, then proceeded to talk about how they hated their own looks and bodies.

Mary Pipher's book *Reviving Ophelia* looks at case studies of adolescent girls falling into depression, eating disorders, addictions, and suicide, blaming themselves for not being attractive or good enough. Whether from cultural pressure and family conditioning or messages from boyfriends, the fashion industry, fitness trainers, doctors, priests, cops, celebrities, and wherever else they come from, this inappropriate and dangerous surrender of instinctual knowledge is at the core of women's disembodied relationship with their own health and fitness.

How did it all become so complicated? When did the simple act of physical activity—the birthright of every human—become the guilt-ridden drudgery of endless stair-stepping? "Forced exercise has all the appeal of a prison labor camp," said Cheryl, a marketing specialist who has been dieting and exercising her entire life.

Granted, our sedentary lifestyles are major culprits in the way we have distanced ourselves from normal daily physical activity. "But who wants to sit on a stationary cycle at night after sitting at a computer all day and then driving home on the freeway for an hour?" complained a 56-year-old writer and editor. "I feel like my butt can't take another minute parked on that damn bike. My kids talked me into one of those rowers, and I won't sit on that, either."

AVOIDING THE LIFESTYLE OVERHAUL

Even though we give a lot of lip service to healthy choices, what's happened in today's society is an obsession with the *wrong* ways to live. People tend to focus on the negative, on everything they shouldn't do. The fitness industry counts on our obsession with lifestyle vices.

Fitness counselors at the Duke University Diet and Fitness Center in Durham, North Carolina, know that overhauling your lifestyle for the long term can be next to impossible without yearly "tune-ups," so they established a return visit policy for graduates of their lifestyle education program. One woman who said that she has been overweight all her life knows that she must maintain the daily grind or she will fall off the wagon. "I have to exercise for 1½ to 2 hours every single day, without fail, and I must always restrict and watch every morsel that goes into my mouth," she said. As one of the lifestyle counselors at the Pritikin Center for Longevity in Santa Monica explains, "It has to be a daily obsession, or they fail. Those who can commit to that mo-ment-by-moment awareness are the ones who succeed."

Fail at what? Succeed at what? Moment-to-moment obsession? Is this any way to live? It is time to completely rethink how we approach healthy eating and exercise as lifetime pursuits. If it is an uncomfortable, deprivation-oriented approach, all we are doing is waiting to reward ourselves with a return to nor-malcy. "If we can modify our lifestyles in small, bite-size chunks instead of the great overhaul," advises health promoter Molly Mettler, "we don't go crazy after the diet or just sit on the couch after a month of step classes. The real rev-olution in changing habits must be motivated from within. We're in the midst of a self-care revolution, and we have to realize that once people are educated with enough options, they generally will find something that suits them and that they can modify easily."

Helping you find something that suits you is my goal in this book. First, however, you must be convinced, deep in your heart, that you are the best judge of what your body enjoys doing and how to do it. Wind your way through these pages and together, I promise, we will concoct your own mixed bag of moveable treats—ways to move you, over and over again.

2

Discover Your Fitness Personality

Before you put on your sneakers and exercise clothes, before you sweat one bit, you're going to sit down and get to know yourself a lot better. You're going to explore the inner you: your thoughts, feelings, needs, fears, desires, preferences, rejections—the whole shebang.

Why? Because every person has an innate fitness personality based on these inner feelings. For years, the fitness industry has coaxed you into burying this personality and ignoring all those inner yearnings and preferences. They told you that the moves you naturally preferred wouldn't work, that they wouldn't improve your health or help you lose weight. That is all plain hogwash. You didn't know that, though, so you learned to ignore your natural instincts. It ended up making you fail at fitness.

Now, it's time to get back in touch with yourself. You see, once you have an accurate assessment of your strengths, weaknesses, preferences, and dislikes, you will be able to make choices that are better aligned with your deepest character traits. This exponentially enhances your chances for successfully following a new fitness routine.

To discover your fitness personality, start by taking the test that follows and reading through the personality descriptions. Then find your Enneagram type on page 26. Armed with the information from all of the self-discovery tools, you'll be ready to discover your movement type, which will accompany you throughout *The Fitness Instinct*. Let's get started.

WHO ARE YOU?

How we respond to stress, how we react to conflict, whether we prefer a gregarious gathering to a quiet tête-à-tête—all of these factors shape our personalities. Just as we have inborn preferences that guide our friendships and career choices, we also have instinctual preferences that should guide our fitness choices. The problem is that many of us are out of touch with our natural inclinations.

The following tests, however, will help you get back in touch.

The first test has been modified from a brain typing method developed by Jonathan Niednagel, an athletic consultant for professional teams and athletes. In his book *Your Key to Sports Success*, Niednagel explains how each of us falls into one of 16 inborn brain types. Knowing about your type helps you understand the best ways to motivate yourself and which innate talents to develop. You can even discover which sport and speed are ideal for you as well as which types of pressure to avoid and which types will challenge you. I've boiled those 16 types down to 4 major ones, giving you a more-than-adequate read on your optimal training and movement potential.

For the following questions, choose the description—"a" or "b"—that you feel fits you best. Check "c" if you feel that the person who knows you best (spouse, relative, friend, etc.) would disagree with your answer. Thus, for certain questions, you may have two answers checked, either "a" and "c" or "b" and "c."

1. a. Higher energy level, sociable
   b. Lower energy level, reserved, soft-spoken
   c. Close associate probably disagrees

2. a. Interprets matters literally, relies on common sense
   b. Looks for meaning and possibilities, relies on foresight
   c. Close associate probably disagrees

3. a. Logical thinking, questioning
   b. Empathetic, feeling, accommodating
   c. Close associate probably disagrees

4. a. Organized, orderly
   b. Flexible, adaptable
   c. Close associate probably disagrees

5. a. Outgoing, makes things happen
   b. Shy, does fewer things
   c. Close associate probably disagrees

6. a. Practical, realistic, experiential
   b. Imaginative, innovative, theoretical
   c. Close associate probably disagrees

7. a. Candid, straightforward, frank
   b. Tactful, kind, encouraging
   c. Close associate probably disagrees

8. a. Plans, schedules
   b. Unplanned, spontaneous
   c. Close associate probably disagrees

9. a. Seeks many tasks, public activities, interaction with others
   b. Seeks more private, solitary activities with quiet to concentrate
   c. Close associate probably disagrees

10. a. Standard, usual, conventional
    b. Different, novel, unique
    c. Close associate probably disagrees

11. a. Firm, tends to criticize, holds the line
    b. Gentle, tends to appreciate, conciliate
    c. Close associate probably disagrees

12. a. Regulated, structured
    b. Easygoing, live-and-let-live
    c. Close associate probably disagrees

13. a. External, communicative, expressive
    b. Internal, reticent, holds things in
    c. Close associate probably disagrees

14. a. Considers immediate issues, focuses on the here-and-now
    b. Looks to future, global perspective, big picture
    c. Close associate probably disagrees

15. a. Tough-minded, just
    b. Tender-hearted, merciful
    c. Close associate probably disagrees

16. a. Preparation-oriented, work-minded
    b. Goes with the flow, play-minded
    c. Close associate probably disagrees

17. a. Active, initiates
    b. Reflective, deliberates
    c. Close associate probably disagrees

18. a. Facts, things, seeing "what is"
    b. Ideas, dreams, seeing "what could be," philosophical
    c. Close associate probably disagrees

19. a. Matter-of-fact, issue-oriented, principled
    b. Sensitive, people-oriented, compassionate
    c. Close associate probably disagrees

20. a. Controls, governs
    b. Latitude, freedom
    c. Close associate probably disagrees

➤ **Scoring**

What's Your Type?														
	I				**II**				**III**				**IV**	
	a	b	c		a	b	c		a	b	c		a	b	c
1				2				3				4			
5				6				7				8			
9				10				11				12			
13				14				15				16			
17				18				19				20			
	E	**I**			**S**	**N**			**T**	**F**			**J**	**P**	

To find your personal type, add the number of "a" and "b" responses in each column and circle the letter at the bottom of the column that has the most check marks. The circled letters indicate whether you are:

- Extroverted (E) or introverted (I)
- Sensing (S) or intuitive (N)
- Thinking (T) or feeling (F)
- Judging (J) or perceiving (P)

What about the "c" responses? They will tell you where to use caution in evaluating your personality type. If, for example, in column four, you checked three "J" responses, two "P" responses, and three "c" responses, you will have to take some additional time to consider your true preferences. If all of your "J" choices also have "c" marked, for example, you evidently think that someone who knows you well would consider you a "P." If that's the case, you need to think beyond how you *want* yourself to be and come to an honest conclusion regarding your true personality type.

Here are brief explanations of the eight key characteristics. Again, you may not agree with every trait or habit described below. If you answered the questions honestly, however, the majority of characteristics will be accurate. From here, we'll look at how your four key characteristics add up and how they help reveal your fitness personality.

Extrovert. You charge up your energy by being around others and staying connected to people, places, and things. You tend to openly share what you're experiencing and can relate to others easily.

Introvert. You restore your energy through time alone and find retreat from others a welcome relief. You do well at nurturing a few very good relationships rather than many acquaintances, and you tend to reflect deeply.

Sensing. You gather your information about the world through your five senses. Your practical nature keeps you in the here-and-now, and generally, you don't attach a larger meaning to events or conversations with others. You interpret matters literally and place a high value on facts.

Intuitive. Your ability to perceive meaning and significance allows you to move beyond the immediate and scan the possibilities for the future. You tend to overlook the down-to-earth details as you activate your impressive imagination and view life from a loftier perch.

Thinking. You trust decision-making that is based on sound reasoning, objective data, and just policies. Your sense of right and wrong helps you take a systematic approach to problem-solving so you're not caught up in subjective emotions.

Feeling. The high value that you place on relationships allows you to balance facts with feelings, moral standards with circumstances, and principles with compassion. Your decisions weigh in favor of harmony and win-win rather than by-the-book outcomes.

Judging. Your ability to be well-organized makes you the perfect project manager. You know how to put forth a disciplined effort to bring matters to completion and enjoy clear, tidy endings.

Perceiving. Your spontaneity and sense of freedom create a great deal of opportunity for exploration. On a team project, you tend to be the one who asks if all possibilities have been considered and all avenues researched. You hesitate to close a project, always seeking a better answer.

WHAT'S YOUR TYPE?

Based on your scores from the personality quiz, take a look at the following descriptions of the chief personality types. Determine how closely your test results correspond with what you know about yourself. Don't worry if you can't relate to all of the traits. Everyone is unique, and individual variations always occur, but for the most part, a majority of the traits probably clusters within your personality. If they're not self-evident, check the description with friends or family and see if they think it's a match for you.

➤ SJ (Sensing, Judging)

This is your pattern if you had the most check marks in columns ESFJ, ESTJ, ISFJ, or ISTJ.

- Puts work before play
- Relies on five senses
- Churchgoer
- Loyal to country
- Finishes the job

- Guardian, safeguards tradition
- Values home, family
- Trusted employee
- Prepared, detailed
- Independent

➤ SP (Sensing, Perceiving)

This is your pattern if you had the most check marks in columns ESTP, ESFP, ISTP, or ISFP.

- Freedom-loving
- Proficient with tools
- Lives for the moment
- Persuasive
- Realistic, down-to-earth
- Action-oriented
- Risk taker
- Entertaining
- Warm and playful
- Optimistic negotiator

➤ NF (Intuitive, Feeling)

This is your pattern if you had the most check marks in columns ENFP, ENFJ, INFP, or INFJ.

- Communicator
- Idealistic
- Optimistic
- Good counselor
- Empathetic
- Warm and engaging
- Visionary
- Lots of possibilities
- Looks for meaning and purpose
- Expressive

➤ **NT (Intuitive, Thinking)**

This is your pattern if you had the most check marks in columns ENTJ, ENTP, INTJ, or INTP.

- Curious, inventive
- Skeptical
- Competent
- Independent
- Entrepreneurial
- Logical
- Wants to excel
- Theoretical
- Alert thinker
- Enjoys a challenge

After taking this test, you should have a pretty good idea of your personality pattern. Now let's delve a little deeper.

YOUR ENNEAGRAM TYPE

The Enneagram is a dynamic personality system based on an interconnected diagram of nine types. Used by psychologists with their clients and by human resource directors in work settings, its origin is a bit mysterious. Some trace it to the mathematical discoveries of the Greeks at the time of Pythagoras, others to the Sufis and Islamic mystics. I think that it goes back even further, to the Ennead, the pantheon of nine gods and goddesses in ancient Egypt.

I spent a month in Egypt as a journalist, visiting the Cairo museums and the tombs of the pharaohs and discussing with Egyptologists the nine specific characteristics of the adventuresome and wayward deities in the Ennead: Atum, Shu, Tefnut, Seb, Nut, Osiris, Isis, Seth, and Nephthys. Their myths constitute the strengths, weaknesses, and unique traits contained within each of the nine descriptions of the Enneagram. It seems that the fundamental patterns of human functioning have been recognized, at least in folklore, for millennia.

The simple way to determine your Enneagram number is to read the characteristics, discuss them with others, and come to an honest conclusion about which of the nine best represents who you are (rather than who you want to be). Be honest. Once you claim a type, you'll find an interesting parallel between your number and your movement personality as you read on.

1. Puritan

Strengths: Motivated by ideals to reform, crusades for principles.
Weaknesses: Moralizing and abrasive, self-righteously dogmatic.
What others think: Improves the situation but can't take criticism.

2. Helper

Strengths: Loves to be helpful, capable of unconditional love, generous.
Weakness: Places others on a guilt trip, plays martyr, hypochondriac.
What others think: Needs to be appreciated and vindicated.

3. Producer

Strengths: Self-assured, energetic, popular, appears lucky or widely admired.
Weakness: Can be exploitative and deceptive.
What others think: Admired for competency but avoided for narcissism.

4. Artist

Strengths: Sensitive, creative, honest.
Weaknesses: Alienated and prone to depression, escapist, emotionally blocked.
What others think: Has creative gifts but tends to be self-absorbed.

5. Thinker

Strengths: Very perceptive, deeply thoughtful, mentally adept, has valuable ideas.
Weaknesses: Can get detached from reality, overly fond of the unorthodox, paranoid.
What others think: Sought after for understanding but cold and remote.

6. Loyalist

Strengths: Trustworthy upholder of authority, cooperative and appealing.
Weakness: Insecure and self-defeating, beset with anxieties.

What others think: Fun to be around, but their fears are constantly testing others' friendship.

7. Dilettante

Strengths: Enjoys doing many things, enthusiastic and appreciative.

Weaknesses: Demanding and childish, superficially dabbling with no consistency.

What others think: Fun but flighty, never seems to have enough, always wants to move on.

8. Commander

Strengths: Naturally assertive leader, confident and protective, instinctive.

Weaknesses: Combative and aggressive, dominates others to get own way.

What others think: Relied on for decisiveness but avoided for violence.

9. Peacemaker

Strengths: Good-natured, supportive and optimistic, fulfilled and peaceful.

Weaknesses: Can be too oblivious and passive, undeveloped, or unaware.

What others think: Helpful presence to resolve tension but doesn't always know what they want.

MATCHING MOVEMENT TO YOUR PERSONALITY

Now that you've gotten to know yourself well, you're ready to take the next step toward instinctive fitness by understanding how movement is paired with personality.

Observations of human dynamics and authentic movement have demonstrated that as you behave, so do you move. Our everyday speech is filled with typical descriptions. Did you ever hear someone describe a big, lumbering, warm-hearted bear of a guy? Or maybe you can think of some frenetic, high-strung, wiry, squirrelly people.

Researchers in sports psychology and dance therapy have found that there is an undeniable correlation between how our brains and nervous systems function and how we move. By just watching someone walk across a room, movement analysts can describe the person's personal history, family experiences, fears, and competencies. They are basically "reading" the intricate linkage between mind and body from verbal, nonverbal, and physical expressions.

For example, Stuart Heller, Ph.D., a Chinese medicine movement educator, can tell if you need more fire, earth, wind, or water, the elemental energies that balance our life force. By simply correcting for these imbalances and asking his clients to try a different gesture or posture, Dr. Heller can help them build confidence in standing up to a boss or communicating with their kids. A Laban movement analyst, on the other hand, will use a completely different set of terms to describe your forthrightness or your hesitancy as it shows up in gait and gesture.

A Feldenkrais practitioner can teach a slight modification to a movement that can make you feel as if a ton has been lifted off your shoulders emotionally and physically. I've also been able to offer similar minor adjustments to habitual movements and help many people change their lives in noticeable ways.

In short, you and your body are one, one inseparable universe of thought-made-visible, emotions-made-flesh, and spirit-made-manifest. As such, it's really pretty easy to see how your personality stores its stuff right in your movement medley.

I've translated the four personality types into four movement types: *Racer*, *Stroller*, *Dancer*, and *Trekker*.

To determine your fitness personality, take a look at the chart on page 30. Use the personality type and Enneagram number that you arrived at earlier in this chapter to help identify which of the four categories you fall into. Also look at the list of traits to help verify the match. Again, not every trait will be owned by you. Some will stand out as obviously yours, and a few characteristics simply may not fit. That's normal; after all, each human being is a completely unique person. On the whole, however, one movement type should stand out for you.

"LET'S CONFIRM"

We'll be working with these movement types throughout *The Fitness Instinct*, and you'll get to know them as if they were your new best friends. Even though one of the basic types will be the one you work with predominantly, after a while, you'll be able to perceive yourself in each of the four types, which is a natural outgrowth of self-discovery.

Now that you know your movement personality, let's play a fun, revealing game. Have you ever found yourself doodling away, kind of obsessed with one

Movement type	RACER ⟶	STROLLER ◎
Personality type	SP	SJ
Enneagram	1, 8, 3	1, 9, 7
Energy peak	Morning	Midmorning
Process	Decisive	Relaxed
Mood	Get-to-the-point	Friendly
Dislikes	Wasting time	Conflict
Preferred sensory input	Visual	Visual/Auditory
Reaction style	Instinctive	Sensible
Work style	Overcome	Converge
Moves	Competitive	Balanced
	Karate	Aikido
	Marching	Belly dancing
	Diagonal	Back and forth
	Throw spear	Throw net
Movement type	DANCER ✳	TREKKER
Personality type	NF	NT
Enneagram	2, 3, 4, 6, 7	5, 6
Energy peak	Later midday	Evening
Process	Spontaneous	Systematic
Mood	Engaging	Withdrawn
Dislikes	Wasting effort	Embarrassment
Preferred sensory input	Kinetic	Auditory
Reaction style	Innovative	Analytic
Work style	Diverge	Assimilate
Moves	Go with flow	Disciplined
	Tai chi	Tae kwon do
	Whirling dervish	Ballet
	Meandering	Perpendicular
	Conceal tracks	Build a trail

particular design for a while? Maybe you're drawing concentric circles over and over on napkins, or perhaps it's arrows or triangles.

The symbols we're drawn to can tell us something about the pressures, obsessions, fascinations, and dreams we're wrestling with from time to time. They can also describe the larger framework of our lives.

Inspiration for this game comes from Angeles Arrien, an innovative thinker and cultural anthropologist who did her groundbreaking work on basic universal symbols and their connection with the ways that we unconsciously express our true natures.

To play, draw the following four symbols on four separate sheets of paper: an arrow, spiral, spark, and chevron. Stack them so that the one you like most

(continued on page 34)

SORTING US OUT

Throughout history, deep thinkers have been coming up with ways to sort people. In older times, these categories were based on observation and philosophy or theology. In modern times, scientists have created quizzes and tests that add a level of objectivity to the sorting.

The fitness personalities that I've created correspond nicely with many of these sorting systems, old and new. If you are familiar with any of them, the following will be of interest.

	RACER	STROLLER	DANCER	TREKKER
DISC	Dominance	Steadiness	Influencing	Compliance
DeVille	Controller	Supporter	Entertainer	Comprehender
Jung	Sensate	Feeling	Intuitive	Thinking
Mythology	Athena	Hera	Dionysius	Apollo
Hippocrates	Choleric	Phlegmatic	Sanguine	Melancholic
Plato	Artisan	Guardian	Philosopher	Scientist
Native American	Fire East/Eagle	Earth South/Squirrel	Water West/Bear	Air North/Buffalo

CHALLENGING YOUR MOVEMENT PERSONALITY

You've learned that almost everyone relates to one of four movement personalities: Racer, Stroller, Dancer, or Trekker. You also know now that particular movements and exercise patterns appeal to each personality type, and that the trick to instinctual fitness is to tap into those movements that are most natural and pleasing to you.

I have to admit that there's a small catch to this theory: If you become too comfortable with the movements that fit your personality and stop experimenting with new ones, you'll hold yourself back. The truth is, it's good to experiment with new movements. Making new neural connections, "derailing" from the usual pathways, and pulling out all the stops—that's how you enter new intuitive territory.

If your only movement endeavors are made in the highly rigid, up-and-down structure of a tightly choreographed step class, what does this say about your current state of mind? Does spontaneity have a place in your life? Do you allow for the unrehearsed or the nonstructured? You should. On the other hand, if you're only given to wild, abandoned, structureless, and formless movement, you need to develop the part of you that would benefit from form and structure.

The following "derailers," tailored for each movement personality, will help you break up old movement patterns and clear your path to instinctual fitness.

→ Racer

Natural tendencies: You love skillful strategy and fast-moving adventures. You're fun-loving, competitive, entertaining, and aggressive, but you tend to become bored easily.

Typical pattern: Forward-driven, fast, and focused.

Derail it with: Non-goal-oriented moves. Take a cue from Strollers, with whom you usually don't pair yourself. Try helping someone else's movement and forcing your own to play a simple supporting role. Learn how to be a guide for blind skiers or hikers, for example, or volunteer as a ropes course trainer, assist as a spotter for a local gymnastics school, take a ballroom dance class, or learn the hula.

◉ Stroller

Natural tendencies: You enjoy creating socially supportive relationships. You play by the rules and are often quiet and orderly. You handle pressure well, have long endurance, and excel in routines.

Typical pattern: Balanced, evenly paced, and unrushed.

Derail it with: One-directional, high-speed, focused thrust. Follow the lead of Racers, whom you naturally try to avoid. Try games like racquetball that can fire you up quickly and become competitive. Swim laps and race against the clock. Add sprints to your walking routine.

✳ Dancer

Natural tendencies: You're persuasive, a great mimic, and naturally gifted. You're energetic, with lots of spontaneity. You hate routine.

Typical pattern: Free-form, unplanned, and disordered.

Derail it with: Structure. Follow the example of Trekkers. You'll groan for the first few steps, but it will help you break through to a fresh new experience. Keep your attention on the form and keep it slow. Build a sand sculpture. Follow a weight-training schedule for six weeks and log your progress.

⌁ Trekker

Natural tendencies: You're reliable and trustworthy. A hard worker, you always finish a job, while never overlooking details. You're skilled at types of movement that require long hours of training and consistent posture, form, and refinement.

Typical pattern: Structured, scheduled, and consistent.

Derail it with: Randomness. Do it wrong for a change. Take a cue from Dancers—the wilder and more spontaneous, the better. Play Twister with small, noisy, messy kids. Start a pillow fight. Wash the dog and the car at the same time, and squirt your neighbors while you're at it. Put on the sound track to *West Side Story* or *A Chorus Line* and imitate a Broadway dancer in the living room. (Okay, you can pull the curtains.)

is on top and the one you like least is on the bottom. Do it quickly; don't put much thought into it. Don't read the next paragraph until you're finished.

Surprise: The real psychology of this test is based on a reversal of what you thought you were doing. Here's what each symbol and its position represent.

→ *Arrow.* Racer: action, change, results, drive, strong, can be a steamroller, no hesitation.

ⓔ *Spiral.* Stroller: receptive, containing, persistent and steady, ambiguous, still, makes no sound unless disturbed, unifying, makes sure that all is attended to.

✳ *Spark.* Dancer: raw, spirited, intuitive, can suffer burnout, smolders indefinitely, enjoys wide diversity, leaves no playground untended, needs reminders to rest and restore.

⌐ *Chevron.* Trekker: patient but plodding, purposeful, enjoys economy of movement, stability, knows how to progress and how to grow.

Bottom choice. You think it's what you prefer least, but it's really what you're most adept at and used to. It's the movement personality that operates naturally within your fundamental base and is part of your core competence.

Middle two choices. The middle is anything but static. These cards symbolize important irritants, or "pebbles in your shoe." Aspects of these two movement personalities can serve as allies for you, helping you incorporate and achieve your first choice.

Top choice. What you thought was most desirable is actually the aspect that you need most in order to balance yourself. It's the movement that you're lacking or inadequately expressing. Perhaps the most challenging type for you, it often lies just ahead. It's a good idea to actively seek to add it to your movement repertoire.

3

Free Yourself
from Old Myths

To reach the area of instinctive fitness that exists deep within each of us, we first must journey through what I have come to call the land of Myth-Fits. The landscape is littered with misguided and just-plain-wrong notions that are responsible for endless cycles of false starts and artificial routines. If you get lost in the land of MythFits, you'll never complete your journey to self-discovery. On the other hand, when you get past these predominant myths, you will free up a tremendous amount of physical and mental energy, along with the creativity and passion to pursue holistic fitness.

MythFits are everywhere. You learned them in gym class. You picked them up from exercise videos and infomercials. They just plain inundated you, so don't feel guilty or stupid for believing them. Most people do.

But now, it's time for the truth.

I've broken these 15 MythFits into two categories based on their level of conspicuousness. Level one contains the most obvious, commonly held notions that have been propagated for years, usually due to some misdirected effort or wishful thinking.

The second level is harder to decipher and requires deeper levels of openness, truth-telling, and investigation. That's because the fitness movement is a modern-day Trojan Horse. Both the Greeks and the fitness industry chieftains employed strategies to achieve their goals, with a focus on winning, not on empowering. They fooled their opponents with deception, creating a fear-based environment.

There are dozens of Trojan Horse concepts within the fitness industry, and one by one, we're going to expose them. Be forewarned, though: This section goes against much of the conventional wisdom that you've heard for years. Get ready to open your mind, adjust your attitude, and turn your fitness thinking upside down. Any vertigo is only temporary. For every revelation, you'll dig a layer closer to the core-level, instinctive fitness that resides deep within you.

LEVEL ONE

Myth: **Weight training will create bulky muscles.**

Truth: If you've read myth busters before, you've probably read a response to this one that goes like this: "Weight training will tone and strengthen muscles for women, creating a sleek, lean look. In addition, women's hormones keep them from gaining bulk." Hogwash. That answer is so out of date that it makes bloodletting seem modern. Challenging a muscle with weights creates a hypertrophic effect, meaning that increases in size go hand-in-hand with increases in strength and endurance.

Using lighter weights and doing more repetitions will probably keep this size increase to a minimum. What's visible is some new shapeliness, definition, and taut curves—a definite attribute for any figure. As for hormones, both women and men have estrogens (female) and androgens (male), albeit in different proportions. Women vary widely with regard to the amounts of testosterone they have: There are Dolly Partons and there are Xena, Warrior Princesses. Weight training will increase the size of your muscles, no doubt about it. The extent to which it does is a matter of your training techniques and heredity.

Myth: **Spot-reducing exercises will shrink whatever area you're working on.**

Truth: I always feel sorry for dogs named Spot when I hear this one—and that makes about as much sense as spot reduction. This is a definite no: You can tone and strengthen various muscle groups, but you can't reduce them.

Reductions in size can, however, occur proportionally throughout the body through a combination of consuming fewer calories (controlling your hunger) and expending more calories (exercise).

Size reductions simply don't happen through rote exercise. In fact, lots and lots of repetitions of the same exercise can actually make your butt or thighs larger, not smaller. After placing people on a 12-week program designed from dozens of popular magazine articles labeled "spot reducers for the thighs, hips, and buttocks," I found that those trouble-spot circumferences actually increased. Women had slightly larger thigh measurements after the 12-week program of lunges and squats. Their jeans were *tighter* at the end of the program. This wasn't necessarily a bad thing, since living with more lean muscle is a tremendous benefit for everything from weight control to preventing osteoporosis, but it certainly isn't what the women intended.

Myth: **Situps can give you a flat tummy.**

Truth: "Flat tummy"—this one cracks me up, too. *Tummy* refers to the stomach, which is an organ of digestion. Exercise doesn't do much for it except maybe compete for blood flow distribution after a meal. So what do situps—or preferably, abdominal curls and crunches—do? They strengthen the abdominal muscles, helping to support your internal organs and protect your back from injury. As far as losing a potbelly is concerned, which is what most "flat tummy" concerns are really about, the fat, or adipose tissue, that sits on your abdomen is best trimmed with aerobic exercise, some weight training, and a sensible, healthy eating program. No fad diets, no deprivation.

That is, of course, if your belly is even worth trimming at all. If it's a sudden new crop of abdominal fat, I do suggest that you work on reducing it, since a good deal of research points to higher health risks associated with new "apple" figures (the name applied to those who carry more weight around their middles versus on their legs, hips, and buttocks). If it's a moderate amount of extra weight that you've carried all your life, however, your health risk is no greater than that of a flat-bellied someone who doesn't exercise. Shift your focus from tight abs to feeling vibrant and healthy, and the "flat tummy" worries will reduce on their own.

Myth: **Muscle turns to fat once you stop exercising.**

Truth: No way. Muscle is muscle, and fat is fat; they are two different types of tissue. Former exercisers sometimes keep eating as much as they did when they worked out and then blame their increased girth on this magical conversion, but there's no such thing. When they stopped exercising, all of those extra calories found their way into their fat cells. The extra flab did not come from shrinking muscles.

Myth: **Stretching, warmups, and cooldowns are "extras" and not always necessary.**

Truth: Warmups and cooldowns are absolutely needed. A good warmup gets your heart, lungs, and muscles ready for exercise. This prevents injuries as well as getting you motivated. Always perform 3 to 5 minutes of easier movements at the start and end of each session. Some aerobics classes will also include static stretches at the end of the workout. These stretches help your muscles recover from the exertion and stay loose and supple. While some classes have you stretch before the main workout, it's better to stretch after, since the muscles have warmed up and aren't as prone to micro-tearing.

LEVEL TWO

Myth: **You must work out at a near-maximum intensity to attain benefits.**

Truth: Now, here's some news you'll really like. A woman who stays active all day by cleaning her house, raking leaves, and running errands is just as fit (if not more fit) than a woman who sits at a desk all day and then exercises her brains out for a half-hour two or three times a week.

Researchers have long proven that your overall expenditure of calories throughout the day is more important to your health than the number of calories you burn during a single exercise session. Heavy-duty aerobic workouts like running are not necessary, after all (that is, unless you love to do them). Activities like gardening, bowling, washing the car, and casual dancing boost your health just as much, and for many of us, they are much more enjoyable.

You see, you don't have to exercise so that you huff and puff with your mouth open, able to speak only in short, infrequent half-sentences. Here's proof: Ayurvedic physical therapist Allan Douillard worked with tennis stars like Martina Navratilova, convincing them to bring their intensity down to a level where they could breathe through their noses. The tennis players resisted this idea because they had never trained that way before. Eventually, through a battery of specific sports tests, Douillard showed them how they had actually improved their performance, stamina, focus, and coordination skills.

Douillard knew that breathing through the mouth tends to inflate only the upper lobes of the lungs, which are connected to sympathetic nerve fibers, the branch of the nervous system that activates the fight-or-flight fear response. Breathing through your mouth prepares your body with adrenaline for an emergency response. Your pupils dilate, blood is shunted to your extremities, peripheral blood vessels expand, and so on. The problem with exercising at this level all the time is that you are consistently dipping into a full-alarm state with every workout. If you work out every day, you undergo the ravages

REAL-LIFE INSTINCTS

When I give talks to a large group, I ask them to get out of their chairs and dance in place to some great rock 'n' roll," says Pat Lyons, R.N. "I have them shake out their arms and their hips and get goofy. Then, I ask them to sit down while I ask a few questions:

- Did you have fun?
- How many of you feel good?
- Do you feel some warmth in your arms and legs?
- How many of you feel like you shook off some fatigue from sitting so long?

"I get them to acknowledge that moving was fun. Then I ask the zinger: 'How many of you lost weight just then?' This stumps the crowd. Nobody lost weight. It's as if all the joy of the movement were drained out of them in that second. They returned to this feeling that exercise is serious, hard work that's all about weight loss."

That association, says Lyons, founder of Connections, Women's Health Consulting Network and co-author of *Great Shape*, is what keeps most people on a failure cycle with exercise and diet patterns. Chronically linked with food deprivation, exercise becomes an unsatisfying "guilty should" instead of what it is in parts of the world that don't have diet and fitness industries: jumping, dancing, moving, twirling, walking, running. It's movement—pure, simple movement, part and parcel of all life. It's not a list of calorie-burning activities, rated according to their efficiency, nor is it a precision sequence for optimizing fat-burning metabolism. It's also not simply a means of achieving "fitness," whatever that has come to mean in this society.

of adrenaline toxicity. One of the side effects, for example, is that cortisol (a form of adrenaline) coaxes "bad" LDL cholesterol onto the walls of the coronary arteries.

When you switch to nose breathing, you inflate the entire lung, including the lower lobes, which are connected to the parasympathetic branch of the nervous system, the branch that calms the body, slows the heart rate, relaxes, and soothes. Through proper nose breathing, you employ both branches of the nervous system. At times, the foot is on the brake; at times, it is on the gas. The back-and-forth fluctuation is a balancing act that your body intrinsically knows how to do and that your mind appreciates.

Myth: **You can't be fit and fat.**

Truth: Oh, yes, you can. Just look at champion marathon swimmer Lynne Cox, whose body fat measures 34 percent. The fitness industry would declare her unfit and moderately obese by their standards, yet anyone who can swim rings around the Arctic circle is certainly an athlete of Amazonian proportions. It's time to look at the new evidence.

For decades, epidemiologists have pointed to their highly publicized studies that link weighing too much with a higher risk for heart disease, stroke, high blood pressure, diabetes, and certain cancers. Weight alone certainly can't account for everything, though, because for every fat person who dies of heart disease, three skinnier people do, too.

Fortunately, another group of researchers decided that it was time to look at the relationship among weight, health, and longevity through another lens. Experts at the Cooper Institute for Aerobics Research in Dallas, under the direction of Steven Blair, Ph.D., surveyed more than 25,000 men who had gone to the clinic since the mid-1970s.

The researchers separated the men into two groups, exercisers and nonexercisers, and lo and behold, they found fatter and skinnier men in each of the groups. Among the exercisers, the heavier men had health and longevity profiles similar to those of the thinner ones. A skinny, nonexercising man, however, had a three times higher risk of dying young than a fatter man who did exercise. The critical factor for longevity was exercise.

What's the lesson? If you're at normal weight or even underweight and you don't exercise, you can expect to live as long as someone who's very overweight but exercise. It doesn't really matter how lean you are, since inactivity is the true risk factor.

***Myth:* You're as fit as the number of chinups or pushups you can do.**

Truth: Fitness tests that include the number of chinups, pushups, and other exercises are based on an 18- to 22-year-old man's experience. Few women or seniors have the upper-body strength to do a chinup—and they don't need it. That type of muscle strength is not used for everyday activities.

Fitness tests should be defined by your own experience: the stamina required to chase kids around five days a week, to work at a thankless job, to rush to pick the kids up from day care or school, to buy groceries, cook dinner, feed toddlers, bathe them, supervise bedtime, pay bills, wash clothes, and get up the next morning.

Spending time at a gym is a rarity among working-class, single mothers. Does this mean that they are never fit? Not at all. It just means their lifestyle doesn't permit them the opportunity to dedicate time solely to exercise. They get their exercise by living. Contrast that with the average multiservice fitness club member, who is single or without children, under 35, and college-educated, with disposable income and a high-gratification lifestyle. In other words, most fitness enthusiasts enjoy certain societal privileges.

***Myth:* You must be ripped, taut, and have killer abs.**

Truth: The fitness industry sure does borrow a lot of terms from the battlefield. We go for "killer workouts." Men and women quest for "drop-dead abs." To describe low body fat and highly defined musculature, you note that someone is "cut" or, better yet, "ripped." The video series with one of the longest best-selling runs in history is the *Buns of Steel* workouts. According to Marti West, a fitness expert and business associate of the *Buns* video dynasty, "It's not the content that sells the program, it's the title, plain and simple."

AVOID THESE WORDS	Warning! These terms can be detrimental to humankind.	
	• Buffed	• Arms of steel
	• Cut	• Abs of steel
	• Ripped	• Killer abs
	• Six-packed	• Abs to die for
	• Lean and mean	• Buns of steel
	• Nuclear hardness	• Buns of plutonium

There are now *Abs of Steel* workout programs, plus *Buns of Steel* 2, 3, 4, 5, 6, and—at last count—7, advertised as the "program of lower-body moves that go where no video has ever gone before." Does that mean that my derriere has to go somewhere it has never been before?

Not on your life. The number of hours spent in routines dedicated to overworking one set of muscles is a mind-boggling time demand that can make the rest of your life unmanageable.

I worry about the lack of humanness in all this. So does Paul Linden, Ph.D., head of the Columbus Center for Movement in Ohio. Dr. Linden, who is a specialist in body and movement awareness education, works with people every day who have armored themselves in a steely, protective case, thinking that rigid is powerful. As a martial artist, however, he understands the difference between true power and powerlessness. He says that the ideal posture is "radiant, symmetrical, free, loving, and balanced. It's one where we have free use of our muscles and can respond to any situation with the greatest efficiency." He suggests that we keep our bellies soft, "breathing naturally like babies, moving our diaphragms easily." When we relax our muscles, circulation and oxygenation flow to all of our limbs.

Myth: **More is better.**

Truth: Most fitness trainers will put you through a regimen based on metered progression—you must increase either repetitions, sets, intensity, or speed over time. But life is not lived as an endless linear expansion. Nowhere in nature is this concept carried out, except, of course, in cancer cells, which are the perfect examples of pathology resulting from unchecked progression. Instead, all biosystems thrive on cyclical growth: birth, maturity, decay, rebirth. Our normal cycles consist of energized periods, fatigue, lapses of illness, recovery, and so on.

Think of how you pass through a typical four-season period. There are bouts of flu in winter, and you fall off your exercise routine. You start up again, sluggish but determined, in spring, just like a green sprout poking its head through the soil. Then some crushing work or school deadline in late spring throws your routine out of whack and you're back in that softer, wiggly state once again.

Stop feeling guilty about these layoffs. They're normal. In fact, they're beneficial. They motivate you and allow your body the rest it deserves. Also,

REAL-LIFE INSTINCTS

Eastern Nepal in November is not supposed to be doused with storms, but everything about this trek was unusual from the outset. Although I had stepped up my exercise routine in preparation for this arduous, high-altitude journey, I didn't realize that most of the energy I would need would stem from a certain psychological hardiness.

Eight other Americans and I dragged our weary bodies behind our tireless and friendly Nepalese guides from sea level to almost 15,000 feet. Although we were urged to pack minimally, it's amazing what you suddenly decide that you can't live without as you prepare for a seven-day solo "vision quest" in the most remote part of the world. Some of the men's duffel bags were well over 90 pounds. For 30 days straight, our strapping, home-grown, Nautilus-toned American guys stood by looking very guilty and foolish while five-foot, 116-pound Nepalese, some of them well into their sixties and barefoot, kept climbing and climbing, hauling all of our "must-haves" precariously in straw baskets.

One day, I tried keeping pace with a sweet grandma who carried her 50-pound sack on her head and plodded up the rocky trail in front of me. She must have been in her eighties. She took a brief rest break with me.

I wanted to give her a gift, so I took some gym shoes out of my bag, ones that I didn't think I'd need anymore since I already was wearing my well-insulated, rubber-soled, high-tech, multilayered hiking shoes. We put them on her calloused, tough, brown feet, but a strange thing happened. She couldn't walk well at all. Besides being cumbersome for her, the shoes did something much more depleting—they seemed to cut her off from some sort of power source.

Stunned and a little disappointed, she took them off and handed them back to me, shaking her head and warning me not to wear the little rubber energy vampires. Patting the ground, she indicated that the shoes blocked the Earth's energy so it couldn't reach her. She gave me a tender hug, placed her pack on her head, and proceeded to climb the mountain before us. Within minutes, I lost sight of my barefoot power *amma* (mother), despite my vain attempts to keep up with her.

once you get your fitness routine to a manageable level that you enjoy, don't feel pressured to do more, more, more. You're doing just fine right where you are.

Myth: **You need self-control and determination to become fit.**

Truth: People who succeed in forcing themselves to exercise are losing a very important part of themselves—and it's totally unnecessary.

Much of our thinking in exercise and fitness promotion stems from the belief that if we try hard enough, exert enough self-control and discipline, and overrule bodily instincts, we will achieve powerful, admirable, gravity-defying results. Real improvement, though, requires a change in our patterns of functioning.

From a functional viewpoint, growth or improvement is rarely achieved by forcing yourself through a well-worn pattern. Consciously trying to change a pattern requires that you try to discern among several new possibilities of action or movement. Even recent brain research confirms that new neural dendrite connections can be fashioned whenever we slog through the mental mud and coax the mind and body to abandon the familiar for a new course of action. Seniors who were asked to dance freely scored higher on mental processing and problem-solving tests than seniors who were asked to simply follow directions in a noncontributory way. If we have driven ourselves through willpower to repeat an action to the point of fatigue, and we persist in this action for months at a time, we severely limit our learning process and our options for joyful, efficient, stress-free movement.

Myth: **You must wear expensive shoes for protection and support.**

Truth: Oh, I'm not going to win any friends in the sports apparel industry with this rant, that's for sure. Every fitness professional and piece of fitness advice states that you should wear "good, supportive athletic footwear"— shoes that look like microwave ovens and cost about as much, too. The truth is, the athletic shoe, in its overpriced, overcushioned, and overblown state, can actually cut off your natural feedback loops for safe movement and energy flow.

Supporting evidence for this comes from both alternative medicine findings and my research on the fitness capacities of indigenous people around the world, particularly in Nepal, North Africa, and the mountain villages of Southeast Asia.

Shoes with six obnoxious layers of neopropylene vinyls and indestructible petro-plastics are responsible for more injuries, not fewer, because they give you a false sense of what your body should do. If you are barefoot or wearing minimal natural footwear, like the native people on the various continents I studied, you safely walk, leap, jump, run, and do everything your body desires because you are receiving second-by-second sensory feedback from the pressure receptors and nerve centers along the bottoms of your feet.

My recommendation: Go barefoot. Start by consciously not wearing shoes for a portion of each day. Work up to the great outdoors slowly, since the soles of your feet need time to build protective calluses. Look for uneven surfaces. Your brain will be stimulated by uneven, unexpected, unpredictable surfaces.

I do feel differently about running shoes, by the way. Runners need good shoes for safety and to protect their knees and ankles, which may not be used to the pounding.

Myth: **Energy is merely a by-product of calories burned.**

Truth: Western scientists have always explained energy this way. You eat food and breathe air, and your body uses both to make "energy." Yet, Western science has not recognized the many other ways that our bodies can make energy. Here are some examples.

- Yogis who sustain food fasts of more than 40 days and water fasts of several days without signs of dehydration.
- Tai chi grand masters who knock over five strapping young men at once without even touching them.
- A mother who lifts the front end of a car to save the life of a child.

After intensive studies with a Korean grand master, Tae Yun Kim, who is one of the foremost qi (energy) masters in the world, I had profound experiences of seeing auric fields and electromagnetic resonances surrounding people, plants, and animals. I honestly felt the way that energy can be pulled into your body from the outer atmosphere. In Nepal, I practiced qigong, energy exercises that allowed me to stay warm for seven days and nights at 15,000-foot elevations in the Himalayas.

I know without a doubt that energy is not a finite matter of calories in and calories out. We can double, triple, or expand indefinitely our capacity for gathering and giving energy just by stepping into a new domain.

Myth: **Fitness is something you can buy.**

Truth: Any program that offers scientific "breakthroughs" that require you to buy the latest expensive piece of equipment or the services of an expert to ensure that you exercise "right" is probably a bunch of poppycock. Every year, there are dozens of unscrupulous fitness books with covers that promise "secrets used by the trainers to the stars." *Callanetics*, a best-selling exercise book and video series, boasted of "toning deep muscles previously unknown," an outrageous concept because every major muscle group has been charted since the times of Leonardo da Vinci.

The selling of fitness reaches new lows through television. Half-hour infomercials push walking programs (videos, music tapes, charts, handbooks, posters) for "three easy payments of $49 each."

Most of these ploys are total scams. I know this hypocrisy all too well from having written more than 15 infomercials (I eventually refused to write any more of them, for ethical reasons). Most celebrity spokespeople are merely endorsing the product because they've been given a lucrative contract. Testimonials are "rounded up" weeks in advance of a show's airing by interviewing potentially appealing candidates, shoving a product in their hands at the last minute, and priming them about selling points. Sometimes a testimonial is videotaped for an hour before a usable 10-second byte is flushed out. The public views a quick-edit sequence of trumped-up endorsements. "Calls to action"—the hard sell to pick up the phone and CALL NOW!—are systematically placed in the script to occur every three minutes, according to focus group research. Viewers are carried along for 28 minutes of the hardest sell in merchandising history.

I started analyzing return rates (the products always have a 30-day, money-back guarantee) and reading the reasons that people didn't want the product, whether it was an Abdominizer, a ThighMaster, a Bruce Jenner Treadmill, a *Stop the Insanity* book and audio series, or one of a half-dozen celebrity walking programs. I also had the opportunity to call 24 people who returned fitness products and hear first-hand about their disappointment. Once again, someone's hopes were set on this latest promise, this new magic device that was going to provide a means of weight control and somehow easily rearrange an entire busy day.

The thing is, you already know how to exercise. You don't need to send your money to someone to find out how. You need only to awaken your fitness instinct.

Myth: **You can have that celebrity's body.**

Truth: This one really, really irks me because it's so very destructive to our psyches. Phony images are propped before the vulnerable American public, pushing them to believe that they can have the body of their dreams if only they follow this or that celebrity-driven exercise video.

Over the past decade, I've received at least 500 letters and calls from people who have purchased celebrity exercise videos. They complain about "poor results despite doing every exercise" and religiously following the routines six days a week. Eventually, they are so bored by the whoops and "Come on! Don't give up!"—the chatty wall-to-wall motivators—that they turn off the TV and look for something to eat. Men and women are disgusted with themselves for not having bodies like the celebrities on the covers.

Deep down, you've probably always known that you'd never look like the famous person doing the routines, so I'm probably not surprising you too much by telling you that their routines won't transform your body. Here's the real surprise, though: In real life, that celebrity's routines didn't transform her body, either. Plastic surgery, hours and hours and hours of workouts, and fancy air-brushing did that for her.

I have worked on fitness videos with Cher, Heather Locklear, Paula Abdul, Cathy Lee Crosby, Kathy Smith, Jaclyn Smith, Angela Lansbury, Richard Simmons, and more. Behind every fitness celebrity is a highly paid, well-focused production team dedicated to one purpose—making the star look good. The team consists of a producer, personal manager, publicity director, scriptwriter, choreographer, sports medicine advisor, and technical director, plus a back-up team of instructors.

Many celebs also have home exercise equipment, a self-care schedule, a plastic surgeon, personal trainer, personal manager, full-time low-fat-cuisine cook, makeup specialist, wardrobe wizard, lighting director, and, when all else fails, an air-brush artist for the cover photo.

Cher, Joan Lunden, Paula Abdul, and Kathie Lee Gifford said they were hounded for years before consenting to make videos. Once these reluctant actresses, talk show hosts, and musicians go through the agonizing rehearsals and overnight weight-loss methods, they must master the tricky knack of cueing dance steps, encouraging viewers, and following a complicated routine, all while appearing lighthearted and not sweating off their pound of makeup. They often say it's the hardest work they've ever done.

Jane Fonda told me that she believed she was on a mission to help women discover the hidden athlete within themselves. Her disclosures of bulimia and body self-loathing were applauded by sympathetic fans. She was credited with having transformed a sick obsession into a healthy pastime. And the tapes kept coming. She made 15 videos in 15 years, creating the largest-selling video library in history. Every year, she seemed to look younger, and the public believed that the queen of aerobics was energetically and metabolically superior. Only the editors of the national magazines watched closely as a tuck here and there, a breast lift, or a face lift became evident.

I interviewed Fonda for this project, feeling that the woman who launched a billion leg lifts should be an integral part of the story. Asked about a typical workout schedule, she talked freely about taking a rigorous, six-hour weekend hike with her husband, Ted Turner, but choosing different post-hike activities. Turner would collapse in front of the TV like any other Saturday baseball fan, while Fonda would go to their exercise room and spend another 45 minutes on the stepper and maybe 45 minutes on the cycle, with some additional time using the free weights. When asked if she thought that was excessive, she said yes, of course. It's the way she handles her eating disorders—they've been replaced by exercise.

As a magazine editor, I've received photos that have been air-brushed, trimming inches off the hips and thighs of the skinniest models and celebrities. One cover photo of a celebrity advertising her "amazing new workout" had more than $1,000 worth of air-brushing, removing lines and wrinkles in her face until it looked like a raccoon mask of white-out. *Esquire* ran a photo of Michelle Pfeiffer on its cover with the headline, "Is this the most beautiful woman in America?" and never disclosed the fact that roughly $1,500 worth of air-brushing was performed on her features to adjust her eye width, round out and expand her chin, make her lips fuller, and correct asymmetry in her jawline.

Besides being just plain deceptive, all of this air-brushing hurts us. We can't help but compare ourselves to these commercially sculpted female representations from magazine ads.

Judith Lederman is president of a large publicity and marketing firm in New York that promotes health products and healthy lifestyles. She believes that watching too much television sets up a paradoxical condition in which we idolize the celebrity image we see, while slouching in a position that makes us larger, less active, more complacent, and further from that image every day.

It's a good thing that there are bright spots for change on the horizon. The Body Shop, a successful beauty company that sells only natural products, has a public service–oriented advertisement that features a chubby Barbie doll and reads, "There are 3 billion women who don't look like supermodels and only 8 who do."

4

Fire Your Bad-News
Chorus

Fitness is your natural birthright. I have no doubt about it, but I'd be willing to bet, hands down, that you do. We're going to strategically eliminate all of those self-sabotaging voices—what I call the bad-news chorus—right now.

You can't succeed at fitness until you do this. People I've worked with who made a healthy turnaround first and foremost transformed their thinking about taking care of themselves. They knew that they had to clean out the commonly held assumptions and ingrained ways of thinking that sabotaged their best efforts.

My medical career included working as a psychiatric nurse. To do this, I was trained in cognitive therapy, a mental yoga or thought discipline. Tailoring the principles of cognitive therapy to a holistic fitness model is a concept unique to this book. This rethinking can lead you directly to a sense of exaltation and freedom with your body. It all starts with freeing your mind from delusions and misguided thinking.

Let's start by identifying these misguided notions. To which of the following do you fall prey? Which don't faze you at all?

Replaying the past. Have you ever found yourself thinking, "My childhood was filled with humiliating experiences in sports and physical education. I'm not about to set myself up for failure again."

You're not alone. Eight out of 10 people I studied described attitudes about exercise that were formed during their childhoods. Many had fond memories of childhood play, but unfortunately, they did not associate that play with exercise or movement. Most thought instead of their elementary, junior high, and high school experiences with physical education classes.

An interesting division shaped up among these folks. Generally, those under 30 were split on the subject. The younger crowd could remember some enjoyable PE classes but could also recall the ones that turned them off to ever trying a host of different sports and activities. Those over 30 described classes that had little imagination and were competitive and fairly negative. They felt that "only one or two excelled" and "were picked all the time." They described feelings of being sidelined year after year, of having only one chance to climb the rope, for example, and then being asked to step aside so the more able-bodied kids could practice. Everyone seemed to vividly recall a comment from some ferocious coach.

The problem that arises from these harsh experiences is that we replay old memories and scripts in our minds; we believe that the dark secrets of the past are destined to shape the outcome of our efforts in the present. Too often, people get caught up in their old narratives and are unable to distinguish current experiences from replays. The lesson in mental cleanup is this: If you're blaming your current lack of activity on some rotten early experiences, you have some forgiving and letting go to do.

Discounting. This one generally goes like this: "I don't exercise because I don't see what good it does." One woman I talked with was a retail clerk at a busy clothing store. Ellen never made time to take a walk after work or on weekends because, she said, "I run around at work all day and don't see any benefits. Why would another walk help me?" She discounted the known benefits of walking, and no amount of scientific proof, documented studies, books, or magazine articles would sway her.

Hers was a classic case of more information not mattering. When made into a mental habit, discounting has a way of seeping into all aspects of your life. Ellen not only discounted the benefits of walking, she discounted the benefits of taking time for herself. In essence, she discounted herself.

Using all-or-nothing thinking. I once heard a well-known fitness expert admonish people for not making exercise a "nonnegotiable" part of the day.

> ## FIND YOUR NICHE
>
> With all the choices out there, how can you find the right fitness pursuit for you? How do you know if it is aligned with your fitness instinct? You can evaluate your options based on these three questions.
>
> - Am I likely to find pleasure or satisfaction from the time spent?
> - Does this activity help me appreciate my body? Does it help me foster a positive regard for my strength, flexibility, endurance, or other attributes?
> - Is the process itself one in which I can remain mindful and aware, or do I have to go numb to do it?

Now, I know the well-meaning intentions of this person, but I also know that this type of nonnegotiable, win-lose, all-or-nothing thinking is the death knell for many exercisers.

Instead of taking this hard stance, I suggest that you look at the flexibility you bring to all areas of your life. Where flexibility flourishes, so does health. Looking at situations in terms of negotiability sets up an adversarial relationship with yourself—just the person you're trying to help! If you adopt a nonnegotiable attitude toward exercise, on those days when you miss a workout, you think of yourself as a failure when you really are not. Don't buy it for a minute—it's all an illusion.

Focusing on the negative. Have you ever motivated yourself with this kind of thinking: "I need to start with a test of how out of shape I am; poor test scores may spur me on"?

I'm going to come out loud and clear on this one: Negative feedback is one of the most serious detriments to positive action. I think one of the more significant findings of the past 20 years took place without much fanfare at the University of Wales, when three researchers looked at children and exercise. They wanted to know what most influenced a child's long-term attitude about exercise.

Remember those fitness tests in PE class? Many educators have long thought that handing a kid his exercise scores in front of 30 other children is somehow a motivational tool. In fact, it seems that it is motivating only for those few children who excel and will someday be elite athletes. For the vast majority who receive negative feedback, the poor scores serve only to decrease any positive feelings about exercising or playing sports in the future. According to the researchers, poor scores "reduced intrinsic motivation." In other words, they bummed out the kids for years to come!

Lesson learned: Don't bother worrying about your fitness level today. Just start moving.

Living for the future. This bizarre yet common advice has been handed out for years: "Just do it now, you'll be pleased in the future . . . So what if you hate doing leg lifts? Someday, you'll be happy you did them . . . Too bad if you hate going to the gym and getting on the stepper. In 30 years, you

THE STEPS TO CHANGE

One of the chief limitations of putting health and fitness advice in a book is that it can be tailored only to categories of people and types of personalities, never to individuals. Thus, the advice is understandably limited. If I were talking with you one-on-one, I'd ask, "How ready are you to enjoy holistic fitness? How ready are you to be your own trainer, to keep yourself motivated? In fact, how ready are you for any of this?"

You can find out just how ready you are to tap into your fitness instinct by seeing where you are in the natural intuitive process of change. These steps are based on research that found that all people progress through five stages when adopting a new habit or lifestyle. University of Rhode Island researchers and psychologists James O. Prochaska, Ph.D.; John C. Norcross, Ph.D.; and Carlo C. DiClemente, Ph.D.; developed the Stages of Change Model based upon their experiences with thousands of people who have successfully made healthy lifestyle changes. According to the theory, you progress through all of the following stages naturally.

Precontemplation. In this stage, you're not even thinking about making a change. For instance, a teenager who is smoking to fit in and look cool and considers any talk about quitting just another nagging lecture is a precontemplator. A 45-year-old smoker with chronic bronchitis who is asking his friend if those nicotine patches are any good, on the other hand, is not a precontemplator. They're both smokers, but the bronchitis sufferer has moved on to the next stage.

Contemplation. This marks the first sign of interest in change. You have made won't have a heart attack like your father did, and then you'll be pleased."

For many years, I joined other health professionals in counseling people to establish healthy habits by getting them to focus on the future. "True, this exercise routine may be unpleasant, boring, or uncomfortable now, but just think what it promises for the future," we'd say. "Endure pain today so you can be happy tomorrow." We'd tell them, "You can distract yourself by doing any number of things (reading, watching TV, listening to tapes) to pull you away from your present agony." Distraction. Living in the future. Not being here and now.

it at least to this stage already or you would not be reading this book. In contemplation, you think about the benefits that change, such as integrating more movement into your life, will offer and about the obstacles blocking your efforts. If you're at this stage, you admit that physical activity is good for you, but you're still stymied by the barriers to engaging in it.

Preparation. In this stage, you're ready to make a committed change within the next 30 days. You're preparing emotionally, mentally, and physically by gathering information and resources. At this point, you're able to list more pros than cons for the change you're preparing to make. You may have tested the waters a few times already, but not consistently. You're addressing the obstacles and starting to understand how to overcome them. Preparers join health clubs and buy exercise equipment. They may even have bought new shoes—they just haven't put them on yet.

Active. Congratulations! You've made the change and are practicing a new, healthy behavior. Social support and sharing the activity with like-minded folks is very helpful, since you'll experience lapses. Nevertheless, your commitment is strong and you get back on track easily. It's not unusual for people to visit this stage many times over a lifetime.

Maintenance. You have accomplished and demonstrated change for the past 30 days. Now the focus is on maintaining and integrating the new behavior into your life. You begin to focus on the benefits of exercise, realizing them one at a time. Look for new rewards. Create solutions to any new obstacles. Build daily confidence.

Well, four years and a couple of thousand interviews later, I discovered that this advice backfires on people. A miserable present does not create a happy future. If you're not skilled at experiencing joy and happiness today, when tomorrow rolls around, you won't have the skills to experience them then, either.

Happiness is best honed through daily practice, and like all practices, it can be performed only in the present time. When you've lived your life for 30 years in fast-forward, it becomes extremely difficult to kick back with a sense of mindful awareness, deliberate joy, and conscious presence.

Pretending, hiding out, and otherwise sticking your head in the sand. "Pretending" is a nice way of saying "acting irresponsibly." Pretending that something or someone else is in charge is the opposite of being accountable for the results. Laying blame elsewhere, passing the buck, and pointing to circumstances are all part of a syndrome of unaccountability.

There's an old saying, a paraphrase of Spinoza's philosophy: "If it's to be, it's up to me." Frankly, you get a lot of support for being unaccountable whenever you hear an avalanche of public health statistics. Not a week goes by without a media announcement about the chief killers of our time, namely heart disease, stroke, high blood pressure, diabetes, and cancer. These diseases loom larger than life, strike fear into our hearts, and present themselves with crushing statistics. "One in two deaths is from cardiovascular disease." "Breast cancer now looms at one in nine." "Obesity results in 300,000 deaths per year." Even though we're told that these are all diseases of lifestyle, with preventable components, the people I interviewed felt that the focus on these grim statistics left them alone and powerless to reverse the onward march of these relentless killers.

It's time for a reality check. First of all, the statistics are warped into a sound-byte distortion. It's just plain junk science to say that 300,000 deaths per year are caused by being overweight, and the breast cancer figure relates only to women at the very end of their life spans, taking into account death and disability from all other causes up to that point. Don't let often-repeated, never-explained statistics bamboozle or sidetrack you. It's far better to re-focus your awareness on what you can do to stay as healthy as you can by becoming mindfully aware of your actions. The things that really kill us—the actual underlying causes—are:

- Tobacco use and second-hand smoke: 400,000 deaths per year
- Poor diet: 300,000
- Physical inactivity: 250,000
- Misuse of alcohol: 100,000
- Microbes (bacteria, viruses, and the like): 90,000
- Toxic agents: 60,000
- Firearms: 35,000
- Irresponsible sexual behavior: 30,000
- Motor vehicles: 25,000
- Illicit drug use: 20,000

Using self-loathing as a motivator. This approach will trip you up every time. People used to think that being disgusted with their present physical conditions could serve as a good motivator to get some regular exercise. It doesn't work that way. Body disgust is short-range fuel at best. Within two or three sessions, the self-deprecating monologue derails your good intentions and can sideline you permanently. You have to start with a good dose of self-love, no matter what shape you're in. I discovered this through listening to thousands of people.

Not only will you be unable to sustain a routine if you are hating your body, you may also increase your risk of injury. Paul Linden, Ph.D., is a specialist in body and movement awareness education. At his Columbus Center for Movement in Ohio, he noted that the constriction and imbalance created by negative thinking interfere with proper posture and breathing, making fitness exercises more difficult and uncomfortable than they need to be.

In other words, hating your body will generate a self-fulfilling prophecy. Negative feelings will interfere with movement and coordination and create a genuinely distasteful experience, which will validate negative beliefs about exercising.

It's possible to consciously create the body state of balanced, relaxed, energized enjoyment from which to exercise. You can release and balance your body, thereby actually improving biomechanics and performance. Focus on opening your breathing, aligning your body for increased balance, and making the flow of awareness through your body radiant and symmetrical.

INSPIRE YOURSELF WITH AIR

Your breath is your life force. Many cultural philosophies of bodywork, martial arts, and movement revolve around refinement of the breath, since they consider the composite of "air-energy-breath" to be the primary vehicle for charging every cell with life. When you take a moment to breathe with awareness, you oxygenate your brain better, and you clear away the cobwebs. Stale thinking has a chance to evaporate. With every breath, you refocus your mental abilities and allow inspiration to return.

You begin inspirational breath exercises by bringing attention to your breath. Right before reading that sentence, did it seem that you were actually holding your breath? Does your breathing seem shallow or deep? Take a big sigh, let it go, and then notice again. Observe the natural, rhythmic quality of your normal breathing. Remember, you're not judging it, you're just observing it. The power of observation itself is impressive; it will change the nature of your inhalation and exhalation.

You often hear advice that you should switch from breathing primarily from your upper chest to diaphragmatic breathing, or breathing from your belly. People often try to restrict the muscle movement strictly to the diaphragm, the large muscle that sits under your lungs and makes your belly move up and down when you breathe.

Despite how often people encourage diaphragmatic breathing, though, it's really not a natural way to breathe. Normal respiration involves the muscles in both your abdomen and your chest. The strongest movement, of course, should come from your diaphragm, which lowers and expands in order for the lungs to fill when you inhale. Then it relaxes and rises, deflating your lungs when you exhale.

Other muscles, however, including various ones in your abdomen, should assist this action. The secondary muscles of respiration are your intercostals, small muscles between your ribs that expand and contract your rib cage. Muscles of the chest, neck, and back also aid in the process. All of this movement assures that your ability to move air is flexible and can accommodate any need, from the peaceful, quiet breathing of sleep to the fiery yogic breath meant to invigorate your whole being.

Once you learn this whole-body breathing, your study of breath awareness techniques can lead you to surprisingly vivid states of energy. True breathing aficionados acknowledge breathing centers throughout the body, such as the pelvis, the back, throughout the spinal column, and in the sinus cavities of the head. They become experts in "filling" different areas of the body with air as they stretch, massage, or strengthen them. They also brighten their mental, physical, and spiritual states with specific types of breaths, such as the breath of fire (*kapalabhati*) or the victorious breath (*ujjayi*).

For the exercises in this book, you will follow your own suitably paced, natural rhythms of inhalation and exhalation. Make sure that you are doing a combination of both belly and chest movement. You won't be holding the breaths, although retention is a facet of yogic breathing that you may want to explore someday.

A simple breath exercise is the "circle breath," as described by stress-management experts Michelle and Joel Levey in their book *Living in Balance*. Developed originally by bioenergy healer Meitek Wirkus, the circle breath focuses on the movement of air and energy around you.

Begin by becoming aware of your breathing. As you inhale, bring your attention to your center, just below your navel, then circle your attention up your back to the top of your head. As you exhale, picture your breath and energy moving down the front of your body and back to your navel.

Repeat the inhalation, circling the breath and flow of energy up from your navel to the crown of your head, then exhale again, bringing it back down along the front to your center. Keep breathing in this circular fashion, with slight pauses at the crown and the center.

With practice, you'll sense how this orbit of flowing energy encircles you, no matter whether you're at rest, work, or play.

HIRING THE GOOD-NEWS CHORUS

Here's how to move beyond those destructive thoughts to a way of thinking that will help awaken the fitness instinct.

Stop your thoughts. Learning to stop a runaway thought right in its tracks is perhaps the single most noteworthy achievement of contemporary humans, since it employs the higher faculties of the cerebral cortex. On a grand scale, being able to redirect the mind to a more mature response lets us halt prejudice, block fanaticism, and avert warfare. On a personal level, it can prevent a small-minded act of revenge, patch up relationships, or even transform a child abuser. Thus, it should also be able to enliven a few healthy habits.

How easy is it to redirect a thought? Body educators talk about the progress they've charted in people who have suffered childhood abuse, violence, or sexual trauma. That panicky chain reaction of negative thoughts can eventually be rerouted in the brain through active therapy, bodywork, emotional release, forgiveness, and other healing modalities. The initial knee-jerk thought of "This isn't safe—I'm outta here!" can dissolve in just three to five seconds with a relaxation response or focused breathing. Thoughts are rerouted from the primitive brain to the higher reasoning centers of the neocortex, where prior lessons can reshape your conclusions. "I'm outta here!" calms down. "I can handle this," takes its place.

Build a new image. This can be done alone, but you should attempt it first with someone skilled in imagery counseling. The form I find most useful was developed by Martin Rossman, M.D., and David Bresler, Ph.D., co-directors of the Academy for Guided Imagery in Mill Valley, California, and is known as Interactive Guided Imagery. It's different from guided imagery in that it doesn't use prepared scripts from someone else. Instead, interactive imagery taps into the powerful images that you already have in your head.

Say that you have a serious resistance to exercise. Interactive imagery would prompt you to form an image in your mind that represents the part of you that doesn't want to exercise. It could show up as anything—a brick wall, a pest, a couch. You'd then be asked to give it a voice and let it tell you why it doesn't like to exercise.

The interaction with the image leads to insight from your own inner world and intuition. According to my friend Terry Miller, R.N., a skilled practitioner of this method, you're giving this part of you some needed attention and learning a great deal from it. You may also be prompted to describe what change you would like and what feeling you'd like to have associated with that change. Can you remember a time in the past when you did feel good? How did it feel to have that experience? What type of image will evoke that feeling for you again?

The next time the urge to avoid exercise comes over you, you can bring forth that good feeling, using the image you discovered and rehearsed. Eventually, you'll learn to expand and deepen the experience and allow the positive sensations to "rewire" your present challenge. You can go forward into the activity with success, as long as you have your feel-good confidence intact.

Power up. When it comes to cleaning up your thinking, you can't be a wimp about it. You have to fire up your personal power as if your life depends on it. Just don't scare yourself into thinking that this will require inordinate amounts of discipline. Try this convenient and friendly trick suggested by Connie Kirk, Ph.D., a leading researcher at the University of Wisconsin, to see how a change in your thinking can reshape your body. She recommends using a "personal power pack" of tailor-made affirmations, created out of your own needs, wants, and desires.

Write these affirmations on index cards. Shifting your thoughts to the positively framed specifics of what you want allows the law of attraction to work for you. Dr. Kirk suggests that you keep your written affirmations ("I have a strong, healthy body." "I eat wholesome, fresh foods when I'm hungry.") nearby. Read them a few times a day and before you go to sleep. This will harness the energy of your inner advisor.

Grow up. Mature. Get wiser. Get over it.

What kind of advice is this to give when we've been taught that suppressing rage can eat you alive? It's the best advice, says Stuart Sovatsky, Ph.D., author of *Words from the Soul*, and he's in good company. He shares that opinion with the esoteric texts of the world's leading religions: the Christian Bible, Islamic Koran, Judaic Talmud, Hindu Vedas, and Buddhist teachings. Maturation requires that we take the high road, move into wisdom, and let the soul's sentiments lead us to a greater possibility of more life. These sentiments include compassion, longing, gratitude, praise-love, forgiveness, and awe.

Count on a higher power. I remember the early days of the holistic health movement, when New Age principles were all the rage. In the forward rush of naïveté and boundless enthusiasm, many people embraced the idea that coating your day with mental affirmations could create any number of blessings, from financial abundance to perfect health. Since then, holistic researchers such as Kenneth Pelletier, Ph.D., of the Stanford Center for Research in Disease Prevention; Joan Borysenko, Ph.D., author of *Minding the Body, Mending the Mind*; and best-selling author Bernie Siegel, M.D., have roundly advised people to avoid that New Age pitfall.

Many of us have seen well-meaning folks put forth extraordinary efforts to change their thinking in attempts to divert a debilitating, often fatal illness such as cancer, only to wonder on their deathbeds if their psychic wills, their powers of positive thinking, were simply too weak to pull their beleaguered bodies back to good health. We've watched people die, needlessly blaming themselves for one more failing. A grievous error was committed as we experimented with the notion that "your thoughts create your reality." There is a core of wisdom that resides within the statement, but you have to wipe away some confusing mist to get to it.

Saying that we're responsible for every illness, every infection, or every cancer that affects us is going way overboard. We are responsible for our *responses* to disease, tragedy, stress, and loss, and therein lies a world of difference.

Half of the people in my study underwent crises that they believed triggered new directions and more balance in their lives. They described brief periods—a few months to a few years—in which crisis seemed to work them over, sort of tilling the soil of their lives. At first, some of them met their crises head on, trying to reverse or alter sad events that were irreversible (the death of a child or mate; the loss of a job due to a bankrupt employer). This sense of opposing the inevitable or unchangeable might seem like healthy fighting spirit, but other studies, in addition to my own, have proven that it does more damage in the long run and is associated with a further decline in health and shorter longevity.

It's far better to accept conditions that you cannot change and work toward a healthier, more positive outlook in the areas you can alter. The old prayer, "Lord, give me the strength to change what I can, the courage to accept what I cannot, and the wisdom to know the difference," is the greatest health advice ever written. If you keep returning to a hopeless condition, whether by ruminating constantly about it in your mind or by doing the same actions over and over, hoping for different results, you begin to encase yourself in a life of perceived hopelessness. Hopelessness is one of the most destructive influences on your immune system.

What positive thoughts do create is a psychological framework in which the rest of the variables can flourish. Your thoughts and emotions are the springboards from which healthful actions can leap.

chapter

5

Cultivate Your
Still Point

Dear Peg,

As a young mother, I'm frustrated about not shedding the pregnancy pounds. What am I doing wrong? I work out with weights for an hour-and-a-half four times a week, I play racquetball for one to two hours four times a week, and I take an aerobics class every other day. But I don't seem to be accomplishing my weight-loss goals. What else can I do?

—Frustrated in Des Moines

When I received this letter, all I could think was, How on earth did she find time to write me? But this letter was really no different from countless others I receive, all asking for the perfect routine that will sculpt a flawless physique.

I get hundreds of similar letters each week, and I'm continually amazed at the energy and time that people will pour into their fitness goals. For the most part, I encounter people who work long hours, take care of families and homes, and do their best to squeeze in exercise, yet they still cope with creeping pounds and spreading midriffs. In their letters, they berate themselves for their lack of success and bemoan the exercise gimmicks into which they've sunk enormous amounts of money and time—the abdominal rockers, rollers, and punchers. They describe in painstaking detail their weight-training schedules.

They include their body-fat percentages, their measurements, and their food dairies. Their letters are fraught with pleas to help them find, once and for all, an end to their frustrating quests for the perfect exercise routine.

At first, I got equally caught up in these quests. When I wrote back, I'd list the weight-training manuals used by professional body builders, describe routines for interval training, and spout off the latest advice on fat-burning exercises. If they were walking at 3.5 miles per hour, I'd advise walking at 4 miles per hour. If they were doing two sets of 15 reps, I'd say to do three sets of 15 reps. Like dozens of other fitness experts, I engaged in this silly game of upping the numbers and avoiding the real issues.

Until I began to question my own sanity.

Most people would write me again a few weeks later with a new complaint. They'd never mention whether the old suggestion had made the slightest difference. One woman asked me what else she could do for her abdomen, when she was clocking 20 miles of running every week plus two hours of abdominal work a day. Two hours of crunches a day! I think if it could, her poor gut would post a classified ad: "Help! New home desired; trapped in a permanent contraction due to obsessive exerciser."

Her letter made me realize that for most people, this more-better-faster crusade had no possible resolution. I finally stopped to wonder what shape the rest of their lives were in. Were they finding time to read books, play with children, visit older people, plant gardens, or watch sunsets?

SLOW DOWN TO SPEED UP

Trying to follow a vigorous exercise routine as if it were one more "must-do" on a list that's already too long is one of the biggest mistakes people make. We try to do too much, and we proceed, zombielike, from one action to the next without a break, right on the heels of a busy workday and squeezed in among dozens of errands and family demands.

When we make exercise just as stressful as the rest of our lives, we fail. That's because we end up feeling just as negative about our fitness efforts as we do about anything else that's stressful. We end up dreading our workouts. In fact, we'd rather do just the opposite: We'd much rather sleep or veg out in front of the television.

Fortunately, there's a better way. Not only does exercise not have to be stressful, it can actually be a soothing break in the day. To make it a calming experience, however, you first must learn to cultivate the still point, the missing link in just about every other fitness program out there.

How do you still yourself? Every culture in the world has explored that question. What follows is my favorite collection of Eastern meditative arts and Western psychological techniques for cultivating the ultimate paradox in fitness: learning to slow down rather than speed up.

Without mastering the still point, you never sustain your most health-enhancing actions for very long. In fact, no significant, purposeful, directed, result-oriented movement occurs without stillness. Think of a cheetah's uncanny stillness before she bolts like a stream of speckled light across the savannah. Think of a martial artist's latently charged stillness before he strikes with ultimate precision. Cultivating the still point allows you to pack your restful moments with condensed energy and unleash your inner cheetah when you make your move.

FREEZE OUT STRESS

For decades now, health experts have been trying to get us to discover "healthy de-stressors" such as decreasing our activity or de-junking our diets. Instead of bringing us calm, these de-stressors have only made us more stressed. More Americans report having less down-time, eating more high-fat convenience foods, and collapsing in front of the tube every night. All good intentions aside, the old action plans for managing stress seem to be ignored the minute they are posted on the employee bulletin board.

Is there any hope?

Absolutely. In and of itself, stress is not the problem; our *perception* of events is the real culprit. One man's dreaded family reunion is another man's picnic. According to new research, most of the old thinking on stress management did us a disservice by focusing on how to decrease the number of stressors in our days—basically, trying to change the scene. Instead, quality programs should focus on changing our perceptions of those events—basically, changing our minds.

There is a peace-loving garden within you that is the source of all good things. The fruit of your fondest dreams will bud and blossom only when this garden is watered and allowed space, protected from trampling, and fed the right combination of nutrients. In real life, that translates into down-time. No phone calls, faxes, e-mails, TVs, radios, or nonstop chatter. The impetus for all good health habits begins with learning to stop, look, and feel this quiet garden within your being.

One of the most effective calming techniques I've come across is called the Freeze Frame. Oddly enough, it has nothing to do with your overworked brain and everything to do with your underused heart. Researchers at the Institute of HeartMath (IHM) in Boulder Creek, California, have collaborated with Stanford and Duke universities to study how natural rhythms between the heart and brain can improve your health and bring you a sense of peace, well-being, intuition, and mental clarity. Now the question is, How do you get this rhythm?

It's easy. Try this experiment. Imagine a highly stressful moment (anything in the past week will do). When you feel tension, stop the negative reaction by leaving that mental mess and bringing your attention to your heart. Recall a warm, loving memory and savor it for a few minutes. Finally, revisit your predicament, but this time, ask "What's a better way out of this?" This brief, loving exercise is actually a profoundly effective, nonpharmaceutical intervention that has been studied extensively and reported everywhere from the *Journal of Advancement in Medicine* and *Psychosomatics* to the *Journal of Alternative Therapies*.

You can easily use this simple two- to six-minute technique to soothe away stress, but you must practice consistently. Do five Freeze Frames a day to master the feeling of shifting and balancing your head and heart.

Throughout history, sages have referred to the heart as a healing force, a voice for truth, a mender of all pain and suffering. Within the spectrum of electrical energy generated by what the scientists at IHM call heart power—sincere feelings of caring, compassion, appreciation, and love—there is a great deal of intelligence and intuitive wisdom.

The heart generates 2.5 watts of electric power, making it 40 to 60 times more powerful than the brain's electrical output. The heart's natural pacemaker is also self-initiating; nothing in the body tells the heart to start or to stop beating.

With each heartbeat, the heart generates an electrical field that transmits to every cell and extends a doughnut-shaped wave outward from the heart's location. Positive emotions such as appreciation and love will extend this electromagnetic field to a distance of 20 feet or more. Your big, happy doughnut stretches out across the room, so to speak, enticing anyone present to either notice your "good vibes" or pout off in search of some mutually miserable company.

Chances are that you have already experienced a glimmer of this higher-frequency energy during your life. You may have called it a dozen different names: a peak performance, flow state, state of grace, epiphany, or loving afterglow. It's not just a state of heightened competency or awareness. It is also a state of ultimate satisfaction and fulfillment—a sense that all is right with you and the world. Sure, there is still plenty of work to be done, but you are at peace with the actions before you.

MORE SOOTHERS

Because different techniques work best for different types of people, I've provided 14 other still-point exercises in addition to the freeze frame. Take a look at "Personal Training" on page 71 for some exercises that work for your movement type, which you determined in chapter 2.

Also, please keep in mind that the skills for slowing down are not mastered overnight, just as the skills for integrating movement back into your life require steady practice. They require diligence, patience, and commitment to long-term growth. Give yourself time. Relax—and enjoy.

➤ Beginner Breath Exercise

Following your breath in and out of your body is the simplest path to the still point. Your breathing will automatically slow down and become rhythmic, balanced, and steady after just a couple of minutes. Place your attention on your breath as it travels into your mouth, down your throat, into your lungs, and back out. Notice how your breath feels and sounds. Don't worry if your mind wanders. When you notice yourself mulling over problems, simply bring your attention back to your breath.

➤ Six-Directional Breathing

I like the way this exercise helps me project my energy and presence. It's particularly good for people who have experienced physical trauma or abuse because it gives them a tool for building their confidence.

Sit quietly with your eyes shut and inhale through your nose, drawing air into the *tan tien*, an area just below the navel. Exhale through your mouth and direct the flow of air forward. Repeat the breath and imagine that you are guiding your expired air down. With each subsequent breath, move the air up, to the right, to the left, and even behind you.

After you get used to this breathing exercise, imagine qualities such as power, love, softness, or strength flowing through each exhalation. Feel yourself expand your energy field in each direction, then take one more breath and guide the flow outward to all directions at once. Doing this before a confrontation or speech can help you find tremendous power and allow you to act from a sensitive, mindful, loving place.

➤ Appreciative Meditation

I learned this heart-based meditation from an old swami during the 1970s. It works well for the same reason the Freeze Frame technique works: Your heart is simply a powerful healer.

Spend about 20 minutes sitting quietly with your eyes closed while you flood your brain with memories of love, appreciation, and gratitude. Recall a time when you felt deeply appreciative of someone. Really feel the warm rush of feelings that seem to flow out of your heart as you recall as many details as possible.

➤ Dzogchen Meditation

This Tibetan Buddhist practice is one of the easiest forms of meditation to learn. Sit cross-legged with an upright spine and let your body assume the strong, restful posture of a mountain. Keep your eyes open, but don't look around. Instead, bring your attention back into yourself. Concentrate on your breath as you inhale, hold for a few seconds, and then exhale.

This open-eyed meditation is ideal for beginners who tend to fall asleep while meditating and teaches you to remain open to the world, growing in compassion and clarity. Eventually, you will learn to meditate by letting your mind drift to that luminous, thoughtless place, but in the beginning, you can either follow your breath, gaze at a symbolic object, or recite a mantra (see below).

➤ Mantra-Centered Meditation

Maharishi Mahesh Yogi has turned Transcendental Meditation into a highly studied art form. He and others have done extensive research on the health benefits of their practice, proving that it lowers blood pressure, synchronizes brain wave activity, and lowers stress hormone levels.

Done for 20 minutes twice a day, the meditation centers on a mantra or a word—in this case, a Sanskrit word—that carries a special meaning for you. Follow your breath for the first few minutes and then introduce a mantra, such as "love," gently into your mind. Repeating this mantra brings you to an inner peace that allows you to transcend the usual run of constant thoughts. Consider your thoughts as passing clouds that drift by. Notice them and let them go. Don't be upset if they keep popping up. The simple act of being aware that you are having thoughts is your reminder to return to the mantra and let the thoughts go. With practice, you will become more proficient at this act of letting go.

Some of the initial experiments on meditation were done by Harvard researcher Herbert Benson, M.D., who believed that any word would satisfy as a mantra. He suggested that people repeat "one" to themselves. I believe, however, that the word itself carries a power and resonance and that you shouldn't pick one haphazardly. I offer you these Sanskrit words because of their beauty, their ancient wisdom, and their heart-expanding power.

- Shakti (energy)
- Lakshmi (abundance)
- Om (unity)

➤ Walking Meditation

When I was on a "vision quest" in Nepal, my teacher, John Milton, told me a story about an old monk who meditated while he walked. With every step, he

---

PERSONAL TRAINING You have scores of still-point activities to choose from. The ones that will work best for you correlate to your fitness personality. Here are some suggestions.

→ **Racer:** Start with a walking meditation and advance to a mantra-centered meditation.

ⓒ **Stroller:** Start with an appreciative meditation and advance to a walking meditation.

✳ **Dancer:** Start with music and advance to a dzogchen meditation.

⟋⟍ **Trekker:** Start with visualization and advance to an appreciative meditation.

quietly murmured "Ma, ma, ma . . . ," a chant to the mother goddess of all creation. Everyone he passed was able to bask in his deep love and respect for the Earth as he trod from village to village.

His walking meditation was a moving form of *samadhi,* or a deep meditation in which the mind achieves states of radiant clarity. Walking meditations are not vigorous power walks with fixed goals of speed, time, and distance. They are mantra-guided, easy movement states in which the mind is able to reach expanded awareness because the body is responding to a very low level of sensory stimuli.

To do a walking meditation, pick a route that you are utterly familiar with and that presents no dangers, safety issues, barriers, or difficult navigation. Avoid areas with heavy traffic or shop windows that may entice you to stop and look. Walk at an easy pace for at least 10 minutes, keeping your attention on a single mantra or positive phrase. As your mind wanders, let the soft strike of your foot on the ground serve as a gentle reminder to calmly return your attention to the meditation. Soon, the cadence of your easy stride, your breath, and your single phrase will harmonize into a steady rhythm, and tensions will evaporate.

➤ Contemplation

Common to many types of Judeo-Christian practice, contemplating life's great questions—Who am I? Is there a God? Where did I come from? What is life's meaning?—has long been a spiritual exercise for the active, alert minds of monks, nuns, rabbis, and seminarians. Because contemplation often involves the weightier issues of the universe, practitioners must learn to allow the process to deepen their awareness of a subject without becoming worried about resolving it. Therefore, contemplation that touches upon the still point requires that you do a releasing of the mind, by letting go and having faith in a higher power, while you turn over a topic from end to end.

➤ Massage

I'm convinced that massage is the single most effective form of alternative therapy that can enhance the quality of your life immediately. The results are so immediate, in fact, that when researchers tested people who had just received a massage, they found that they had higher levels of immunoglobulin A, an infection-fighting substance produced by the body, in their saliva within minutes. To maximize the benefits of massage, commit to having one twice a month. The healing power of touch creates a meditative state; increases the flow of energy, blood, and lymph; relaxes muscles; improves range of motion; and influences levels of serotonin and endorphins, brain chemicals that contribute to a positive mood. That's all in addition to making you look and feel great!

➤ Nature

Spending time in a beautiful, natural setting supplies your senses with a variety of gifts. You bathe your eye's rods and cones in the most healing colors: greens, blues, and earthy browns. Your ears take in the natural sounds of birds, insects, streams, and wind. Your nose gets a break from the out-gassing of various petrochemicals from such things as carpets, paints, plastics, and artificial materials in buildings and homes; instead, you inhale the clean scent of the great outdoors.

You should definitely find an area near your home where you can enjoy some peaceful solitude without interruption. In addition, deepen your appreciation of nature by reading some of the finest naturalist writing that exists: stories by John McPhee, tales of Thoreau's daily walks through the woods of New England, or the ponderings of John Muir as he recharged his energies in redwood forests.

➤ Visualization

Many people have profound experiences with this one-minute visualization known as the workshop or the retreat. Read through the following script for the first time, then practice it in your imagination, seated and with your eyes closed. The workshop allows you to retreat from a busy day or a stressful moment and explore a gloriously peaceful and richly comfortable inner world in which you can generate new ideas or solutions.

Picture yourself walking down a path. Take a few seconds to place yourself in the landscape that you find most comfortable and most beautiful. Maybe it's a lush, green forest or an open field. Perhaps you have a vista overlooking something grand and scenic.

Now picture an appealing building just ahead. This is your own re-

treat center, a sort of playful workshop for you to come to and be completely yourself. Take a few seconds to imagine what it looks like. It's custom-built completely to your liking, with plenty of light, windows, and gorgeous furnishings in your favorite colors and textures. The central area is stocked with everything you'd ever want—books, food, toys, games, musical instruments, gadgets, and whatever else pleases you immensely.

Picture yourself resting comfortably in this room, enjoying your solitude for this minute and doing just what you like. Rest easily in this peaceful environment and sense the joy, security, and power that you gain just by being here. When you're ready, slowly depart from your workshop or retreat center by closing the shades, locking the door, and heading down the path again. You know it's always there for you, stocked to the brim with everything you need to restore your strength and creative energies. You know that you'll be back. Leave with a deep appreciation that you have this place within you.

➤ Clearing and Grounding

This wonderful technique from members of the Esalen Institute in California quickly dissipates all thoughts and distractions so that you may gather your strength, confidence, and energy in a more focused manner.

Start by imagining a protective bubble wrapping itself around you, keeping all distractions from you for a brief period. Take some deep breaths while you imagine the bubble reaching from your feet to a space just above your head. Next, place your attention at the base of your spine by imagining a beam of energy going from there through the bubble below your feet, down through all the layers of the Earth's strata, and finally connecting with the Earth's core. Let the energy of the core slowly move up, filling your feet and traveling up your legs and into your belly, drawing up the rich, colorful energies of the Earth. Feel the energy warm your center. As you ground to the Earth, breathe deeply and naturally. Finally, let the rising energy of the Earth's core warm your trunk and your heart and extend out through your limbs to your hands and feet. When the warm, relaxed sensation extends throughout your body, take a final breath, release the bubble, and enjoy renewed vigor from this simple exercise.

➤ Altar Tending

In India and throughout the East, people practice devotional prayer or meditation in front of an altar. In some villages, the altars are small public shrines, or *stupas,* that are festooned with flowers and incense by passersby. In the home, the altars are sites for lively interactions with one's chosen deities. To do a *puja* means that you spend some time in front of the altar rearranging the objects, cleaning it, or decorating it with fresh flowers, sometimes burning colored candles and incense. After that bit of housekeeping, you enter into a heartful connection with the higher source represented by the altar, focusing on your hopes, prayers, and intentions for the day; your blessings for others; and your gratitude and appreciation.

I became enchanted with the tradition of tending an altar bedecked with everything that carries sacred meaning in life. To me, it made perfect sense to keep some small part of a church or temple right in our own homes. Combining elements of puja with lessons from Native American teachers about hearth tending and keeping earth shields, I offer you this charming and sweetly rewarding activity for your home.

Consider making a home altar and tending it on a daily basis. First, claim some space and make an agreement with others in your home that this is yours and yours alone, not to be played with, added to, or subtracted from. You won't need much space. The top of a dresser, a small table, or the corner of a room will do.

Next, gather tokens that carry fond memories, such as photos of loved ones, small gifts, pieces of stone or jewelry, or pressed flowers from a bouquet. I've seen altars with treasures from childhood such as simple drawings, pieces of old toys, locks of hair, and cloth dolls.

After you've made a collection that represents your present dreams and focus, work with the idea of centrality. This means that on a day-to-day basis, you move certain objects from the periphery to the central position as symbolic representations of what you're working on. A woman who wanted to quit smoking placed a broken cigarette in a crystal bowl right in the center of her altar. Centrality has to do with your focused energies. As certain goals or issues resolve, replace the token with other items representing more pressing needs.

An altar becomes a living presence when you enliven it with your imagination and place your current concerns in the central spotlight. In no time at all, your altar will serve as a visible memory jogger for your fitness intentions.

➤ Music

Science now confirms what musicians and troubadours have always known: Music can send a healing and sympathic vibration, soothing an aching heart and lifting your spirit. In research on living cells, scientists found that the sound of a C note from a tuning fork lengthened the shape of the cells. An A note changed their color, and an E note made them spherical.

We may think of music as something we play, but actually it is a sequence of vibrations that play us, reducing pain, stimulating the immune system, and boosting energy. Experiment with various musical sequences while working, doing housework, relaxing, or exercising. Notice the effect that each has on you.

Today's fascination with world-beat music celebrates the universality of rhythms and melodies. This music is felt in a freer, more spontaneous way throughout your body. Not only will it enhance your experience, it may even harmonize your mental, physical, and emotional energy. Try some of these powerful pieces.

- Theme from *The Mission*, by Ennio Marricone
- "Adiemus," from Adiemus
- Score from *The Piano*, by Michael Nyman
- Main title theme from *The Last Emperor*, by David Byrne
- "Sail Away," from Enya
- "Sweet Lullaby," from Deep Forest
- "Serenade at the Doorway," by Ann Mortifee
- "Tulku: Season of Souls," by Jim Wilson

➤ Love and Belonging

Love not only makes the world go 'round, it also makes you healthier and happier. Emotional connection can serve as a catalyst for enhancing your immune system and reducing your risk for heart disease, stroke, high blood pressure, and certain cancers.

One of the first researchers to document the connection between a loving heart and a healthy body was Stephen Sinatra, M.D., a cardiologist, bioenergetic practitioner, and director of medical education at Manchester Memorial

Hospital in Connecticut. Dr. Sinatra's work has been echoed by heart researcher Dean Ornish, M.D., who uses a support group format at his Preventive Medicine Research Institute in Sausalito, California, to help patients overcome isolation and loneliness.

Living with social isolation is like being a caged grey wolf, separated from its pack and constantly looking over its shoulder, experiencing a nagging fear of being alone, vulnerable, and without connection or belonging. Breaking the isolation requires cultivating skills for identifying your feelings; communicating them in open, nonblaming ways; listening with the intent to understand another's viewpoint; and validating that viewpoint. Practicing these skills for simple intimacy may help form the first bonds.

Fear of isolation is not always a social dilemma, however. Often, once a degree of comfort and safety is reached with loved ones, the next layer of the onion is peeled back, and you have a chance to confront existential fears, those fears of being a meaningless speck in the universe. This level of fear and isolation is comforted only by religious, spiritual, or philosophical pursuits. According to death-and-dying consultant Amy Harwell, "Being prepared to die allows you to live more fully."

chapter **6**

Awaken Your
Seventh Sense

An old, wise woman in Chicago taught me my most precious lesson ever—
how to listen to my intuition.

I sought her advice because I had been having one strange experience after
another. Once, for instance, I was lying on my bed, waiting for a car full of
friends to honk in front of the house. I rose from the bed, went to the window
to see if they were there, turned to go back to the bed, and stopped dead in my
tracks, staring at my entire body resting there. The awareness of what was occurring zapped through me, and suddenly I was snapped back into my body as
if I'd been shot from a slingshot. Later, I realized how unusual this dream was
because in it, I had a complete view from the window of all that was happening
outside. I saw a fire truck sitting in the driveway and my neighbors gathering
around it—events that I was able to confirm later.

Another time, for no apparent reason, I excused myself from a dinner party,
went to the hospital, and waited in the lobby. I went because I simply couldn't
silence the inner nudge to get up and go. Within minutes, a friend went by in a
wheelchair, his leg in a splint. When he spotted me, his face paled, and he explained that he had just been wishing that I could be there.

On many other occasions, I would hear or sometimes sense this inner voice
and not heed it. I was often frustrated by it, not really knowing whether I
should follow through. Eventually, with the wise woman's help, I grew to trust
the voice and know the difference between my own anxious mental chatter and
that relentless gut feeling.

REAL-LIFE INSTINCTS

Suzette was a working woman in her late twenties whose boyfriend couldn't accept her weight. He constantly pointed out photos of models and girls with waiflike looks, believing that he was motivating her to lose weight. Not only did she chronically diet to please him, she also posted the photos on her refrigerator.

To tap into her fitness instinct, Suzette had to replace the mental scripts that ran through her head every time she looked in the mirror. She had to realize that her boyfriend's words were nothing more than a scripted response from a make-believe world of advertising and fashion images. Back in college, Suzette had been an avid soccer player. She knew she had to return to her love of sports, surround herself with friends who were active and less concerned about their looks, and generally regain her happiness through self-acceptance and healthy activity.

For Suzette, transferring authority back within herself was a unique game plan, assisted by some work in guided imagery. She was able to vividly recall the high points in her life—when she felt safe, joyful, competent, and alive. One particular memory proved tremendously useful: a celebration with friends after a soccer game, in which the winning wasn't as glorious as the camaraderie among the players and the feeling that all was right in the world.

Suzette uses this image and its corresponding heart-warming sensations as daily reminders of what really makes her happy. She was able to unhook from the mindset of "never too lean," generate a still point that brought her immense comfort and confidence, and remind herself that the responsibility of a healthy, fit body was hers alone.

To tap into her fitness instinct, Suzette says that she only had to perform a quick body scan. Just figuring out what she was feeling in the moment, rather than assigning herself one more "should do," allowed Suzette to bypass a cyclical routine of punishing herself with abusive exercise. As she explains, "The war with my body is over. I'm not running away from it anymore. I get to live in it and count on it—and enjoy it!"

I'd like to pass on to you what she taught me.

You are no doubt familiar with the five senses: sight, touch, hearing, smell, and taste. The information we receive through our senses guides our actions, shapes our thinking, and forms our opinions. In addition to your five physical senses, you were born with intuition, your sixth sense.

There are times when your intuition is irrepressible, such as whenever you insist, "I don't know how I know, but I just do. Trust me." Most of the time, however, these intuitive hits come in discreet and quiet ways, gathered from physical sensations, quiet hunches, dreams, and pieces of memories entwined with mental wanderings. Intuition flourishes when we pause, notice, and listen a little more deeply. Intuition is a birthright we all have, and it's sharpened by learning how to decode the information that resides within our brains and bodies.

Awakening and developing your intuition starts with a deep appreciation of how your mind and body function as a harmonious unit—informing, warning, and sensing in subtle ways. This appreciation is also the gateway to your seventh sense, your fitness instinct. Our bodies are normally guided by this movement instinct, which begins the moment the life impulse enters a living creature and stirs throughout its life span.

I discovered this seventh sense when I experienced how the body, when unleashed from previous conditioning and judgment, has an innate wisdom about just what it needs or what it should do. Just as you must open yourself up to different ways of listening to tap into your sixth sense, you need to explore your connection with your body in new ways to reach your body's movement instinct. Here's the four-step process that will take you there.

TRANSFER AUTHORITY BACK TO YOURSELF

Too many people let others "own" their bodies. They let spouses tell them how much weight to lose, mothers-in-law tell them how much to eat, and doctors tell them how much to exercise. To unleash your fitness instinct, you must ignore all of these outside sources of input and look deep within yourself. There you will find an internal source of motivation. Some may call this source an inner advisor, God, the Source, the higher self, or Tao. When you listen to this inner voice, you develop body authority, the confidence and inner power that come from knowing that you're the one in charge of your body and its well-being.

(continued on page 84)

HOW INACTIVITY BECOMES A HABIT

I've often said that we don't really have a problem with creeping obesity in America, but rather a problem with creeping inactivity. We aren't born couch potatoes. It happens slowly, insidiously, over decades. The stages of containment start shortly after we are born.

Stage One

Infants have a vast repertoire of movements. When you talk with them face-to-face in a loving tone or massage their little limbs, they exhibit a rhythmic, symmetrical baby dance. It's quite charming to watch and reminds me of the cobra dancing to the Hindu's flute.

Once babies start scooting, however, they find themselves encased in a world of bumper guards and pillow barricades. The containment walls go up for safety's sake. Let's not fool ourselves, however: They exist more for the sake of convenience than for safety.

Stage Two

From late infancy to age three, a child exhibits the fitness instinct in its purest essence. The instinct to move is unbridled at this age, and the lack of self-critiquing inhibitions allows the child to experiment with every type of movement, from dynamic to languid and from cautious to rhythmic.

On close observation, you can see a wide array of yoga postures in children's natural selections of movement. They perform spontaneous plows, cobras, squats, and headstands until they collapse, sound asleep, in a surrender pose, also appropriately called the child's pose. Young children will also invert themselves regularly, standing on their heads on couches or tumbling on pillows. Researchers believe that they're stimulating the nerve endings along the vestibular system in the inner ear, a necessary movement for the maturation of the emotions and the brain. Do kids know they're doing that? No, they're just having fun!

Yet, in the later months of a baby's first year and beyond, an array of motion-limitation devices shows up. Six-month-olds are placed in jump-up swings suspended from doorways. Tiny children are often left hanging in these self-propelled baby bungees until they collapse into an exhausted heap. Infant seats give way to car seats and strollers. Another method of semicontainment is the infamous toddler roller-scooter, which usurps precious crawling time with frenzied upright motion.

Stage Three

Teaching children to impose limitations on themselves is the third and saddest step in the stopping of movement. In this stage, we go from restricting children with external devices to asking them to be their own immobilizers. It's easy to understand, therefore, why this is a time of great fidgeting—a leaking of pent-up energy that simply cannot be fully contained in 3- to 12-year-olds.

Verbal scolding and commands are constant. Grade-school teachers spend half their time trying to get kids to stay in their chairs, uttering pronouncements such as "Don't get up without permission" and "Don't leave that table until I say so." Parents go crazy trying to get kids to sit still—"Stop squirming!" they admonish. Being asked to sit for prolonged periods at dinner parties, church functions, restaurants, and adult ceremonies is agonizing for children whose bodies are begging to explore.

Stage Four

By the time they reach age 13 or 14, most kids have learned how to sit still. After eight years of grade school and with four years of high school ahead, most teenagers acquiesce to the cultural norm and give up. In fact, lethargy starts to replace natural enthusiasm, and parents begin yelling at their teenagers to sit up straight. The ubiquitous adolescent slouch is part of the collapsing body dynamic that speaks of resentment and rebellion.

Stage Five

Adulthood, for most people, is the crowning achievement of learning to be still. You drive to work, then sit at a computer or behind a desk. You come home and sit in front of the TV or a computer again. Inactivity is a way of life for most people.

Body authority, sometimes called body sovereignty, is a concept used by therapeutic bodyworkers when they are helping victims of sexual abuse or violence recover their autonomy and power. You needn't be a victim of abuse, however, in order to suffer a loss of body authority. Both popular culture and the fitness industry offer plenty of opportunities to siphon it off. So many of us have utterly abandoned any sense of self-authority when it comes to exercise that we have forgotten how and why to move.

Taking back authority is not easy these days. We're bombarded with so many medical findings, research studies, and so-called breakthroughs that we often wonder what really helps, what actions to take, and what sources to trust.

I am not saying that transference of authority is always inappropriate. Obviously, when we are learning a skill that we haven't yet mastered, depending on expert advice adds to our knowledge. Yet, we can't really break the pattern of automatically deferring to experts and other people unless we become aware of the moment of self-effacement and actively replace the automatic response. The next time you consult someone about anything, pause and ask yourself, "Is this an appropriate time to depend on an external authority? Do I need expert advice, or is this well within my domain to figure out and choose?"

STAY PRESENT IN THE FITNESS MOMENT

"I can teach an entire aerobics class and somehow have no awareness of being in my body. My mind is wandering the whole time, and at the end of the workout, I actually feel vacant, as if I haven't been there. Then I take a couple of classes taught by somebody else and get on the Stairmaster for an hour. It takes all day sometimes before I feel like I've exercised and really worked up a sweat," says 28-year-old Laurie.

Some people may find Laurie's checked-out feeling appealing. Since workouts are usually a drag, what's wrong with mentally deserting for the hour? Plenty. The way to enjoy something is not by shutting down until it's over. Reinforced escapism leads to utter avoidance. Performing workouts that they detest is the chief reason that people drop out of their fitness commitments.

Even worse, this escapism may hurt our health. Stress comes at us from so many different angles these days, such as noise pollution, fatigue, and traffic, that our bodies can't really differentiate among various types of stressors.

When you're in a state of disembodied exercise, you have triggered the stress response. Your body is in a heightened state of preparedness, expecting you to demand a sudden, explosive, powerful call to action. In an ideal world, you would be able to make a mad dash and make good use of your increased heart rate, higher blood pressure, enhanced blood flow, and dilated pupils. You would explode into action and then take a much-needed rest, allowing all systems to return to normal. Instead, you may be prolonging the damaging stress response by robotically working out on a stair climber as you distract yourself with a personal stereo, TV, or book.

You end up inflicting unnecessary physical wear and tear. You ignore unnatural jolts, wearing out your joints and pounding the heck out of cartilage. I know many marathoners who could only train in a disembodied state, and today they are facing total hip and knee replacements because they trained their minds to check out, disengage, and ignore discomfort and repetitive shock.

This concept of embodiment doesn't apply just to times of exertion, of course. After several hours of being entranced in front of a computer, you'll find that your body is achy, tense, and unhappy; you've become disembodied. The goal is to have a sense of your body's disposition throughout your waking hours. To do that, you need to check in with yourself at least once an hour. Ask yourself the following questions.

- How's my posture?
- How long have I been in one position?
- Do I have any sore spots that I've ignored for the past hour?
- How's my breathing—smooth and full or shallow and jerky?

Simply asking those questions initiates the re-embodiment process. Make sure that you don't berate yourself for being "out there" again. It's absolutely normal to flow in and out of awareness. What you accomplish by checking in more frequently is to shift the ratio of time so that the majority is spent embodied rather than disembodied. The benefits of doing so are greater effectiveness, clarity of mind, focus, inner calm, and improved health.

DO A BODY SCAN REGULARLY

Has this ever happened to you? You finish a long, hard day at work and say to yourself, "I should go to the gym." Or maybe, on the morning after a late night, you wake up tired but think, "I should go for a run." Thinking of exercise as a "should" leaves you with only two choices. If you don't exercise, you not only blame yourself for making the wrong choice, you also reinforce a negative pattern of "should, but didn't," and start to label yourself an exercise failure. If you do exercise as a "should," you end up hating every minute of it.

The body scan is a quick and easy way to take the dreaded "shoulds" out of exercise. It detours the usual ways that you think about exercise and tunes in to what you really need. It works on the principle that there are basically four different physical states of being: fatigued, tense, languid, and dynamic. Figuring out which of these four states you're presently in is your ticket to your fitness instinct.

THE WISDOM OF ALL FOURS

The optimal time for crawling is 4 to 12 months of age. This is when a baby's developing brain is tackling a mind-boggling number of tasks, including organizing sensory stimuli, language initiation, and spatial awareness.

The problem is, many of us didn't get a chance to crawl enough when we were toddlers. Nifty baby entertainment devices such as walkers allowed us to propel our bodies by paddling our toes against the floor. Such scooters replaced a significant amount of time that we normally would have spent on all fours.

The benefits of crawling have been well-documented by pediatric physical medicine specialists. The cross-crawl pattern (basic crawling on all fours) is a co-ordinated rhythm of bilateral, opposite-sided arms and legs moving together. Bi-hemispheric brain stimulation occurs through the steady repetition of right arm-left leg motion alternating with left arm-right leg motion. The brain, spine, and the rest of the nervous system are bustling with messages conducted in a two-way flow as sensory impulses travel from the limbs up the spine to the brain, and directional orders from the brain move down the spine to the muscles of the limbs.

Your practice: Take some extra time crawling around as you look for your shoes in the morning. Or mimic the dog by "chasing your tail" on all fours. Crawl for a few minutes each day. If anyone asks what you're doing, say that you're stimulating the left and right hemispheres of your brain. Then have a good laugh.

To do the body scan, check your physical status. Close your eyes, take a breath, exhale slowly, and scan your body from head to toe. What best describes your energetic state?

As you scan, you'll get in touch with the truth of your present condition. You'll realize that there are no "shoulds" in there; there is only "what is so." The "shoulds" of conventional exercise thinking are uncreative, ineffective, habitual responses, inadequate for determining what is really called for. The body scan will let you accurately sense your physical need and choose a suitable antidote. Movement is good medicine, but only when the choice of movement fits the physiological need.

To simplify matters, I've interpreted the four physical states as too tired, too wired, too uninspired, and too mired. Here's how to tell which state you're in and which fitness activities best address your body's needs.

Too tired. If your entire body is achy, tired, and limp, you need to replenish your energies. You require gentle movements that act as turbines, recharging your batteries. Go to "Energy Generators" on page 88.

Too wired. If you have sufficient physical energy but you're feeling tense and wired, then you need to de-stress and unwind, not engage in more heated-up exercise that will create more tension. Your muscles need to completely relax and release toxins and by-products of metabolism before they engage in efficient, satisfying exercise. Go to "De-Stressing Soothers" on page 88.

Too uninspired. If you have sufficient physical energy but are feeling dull and languid, you need a movement pattern with some creative fire to spark your life force. Your energy is available, but it is stagnant, like a body of water without a current. "Creative Sparks," on page 89, will electrify and zap a wave of energizing movement throughout your entire being—mind, body, and spirit.

Too mired. If you've been entrenched in a routine that is driving you batty, you are ready for "Moveable Treats" (see page 89). These are the times when being stuck in a rut hasn't really drained your life force. You are itching with energy to break out. Moveable treats are activities that use that pent-up energy while giving you a delightful break from routine.

Once you've done the body scan and figured out which of the four physical states you are presently in, choose from the following fitness moves, based on what your body needs.

When you're too tired:

ENERGY GENERATORS

The old thinking in fitness said that if you're tired, you need to generate energy with some exercise. I don't believe that anymore. I've talked with too many people who've pushed themselves too hard, thinking that they could shed their fatigue with some high-adrenaline aerobics.

Energy generators are your answer to exhaustion. Excellent for getting you in touch with your energy source (known as qi or chi, prana, or life force), generators do not draw from your energy reserves. Instead, they add to them. Here are some examples.

- Swinging a bat or golf club
- Jumping on a minitrampoline
- Rocking or swaying
- Playing with a hula hoop
- Practicing the Asian movement art of tai chi
- Jumping rope
- Doing yoga poses

When you're too wired:

DE-STRESSING SOOTHERS

These delightful excursions are designed to eliminate the harmful effects of chronic stress. Each of them will release tension, help you unwind, stretch your muscles, and open your joints. They also help you increase circulation, which is vital for removing toxins and by-products of fatigue or anxiousness. The following movements and soothers will play a crucial role in elongating your muscles, oxygenating the tissues, and helping the various systems of elimination perform at their optimum level.

- Stretching
- Rolling on a body ball
- Using herbs and tonics
- Walking meditation
- Using visualization
- Doing relaxing yoga
- Practicing the Japanese martial art of aikido
- Moving to music
- Getting a massage

When you're too uninspired:

CREATIVE SPARKS

Wild, fun, and electric, creative sparks are designed to sweep the cobwebs from your mind, body, and spirit. These rhythmic marvels are tried-and-true doldrum chasers for enhancing creativity, innovation, and spirited breakthroughs. I've found that they are excellent before brainstorming sessions. Creative sparks are also the movement elixir, helping you restore lightness and energy after an arduous mental task.

- Belly, jazz, salsa, or swing dancing
- Hitting golf balls at a driving range
- Gardening
- Attending dog-training classes
- Doing spontaneous movements
- Practicing the wave
- Crawling
- Playing improvisational movement games
- Doing the Head-to-Toe Kickstart program (see page 94)
- Building sand castles
- Participating in world-beat dance classes

When you're too mired:

MOVEABLE TREATS

Do these when you're bursting with good energy but require an outlet for nudging your body into new challenges. Moveable treats are designed to restore a sense of play, sports, creativity, humor, adventure, lightness, frolic, and youthful vigor. These treats are the most extroverted of all the moves. Dancers like to hang out here the most, but Trekkers, Strollers, and Racers should give them a try when they're seeking a challenging experience.

- Kickboxing or martial arts
- Cycling or Spinning
- Taking a nature hike
- Body drumming
- Running interval sprints
- Orienteering (trail reading)
- Taking points-of-interest city walks
- Kayaking or river rafting
- Rock climbing or bouldering
- Inline skating
- Surfing or water polo

FITNESS AWAITS

As you transfer authority and become present during movement, proficient with the body scan, and comfortable with your derailing activities, your fitness instinct will grow. Remember to keep working on the skills you've already learned. Reading once through the MythFits in chapter 3 doesn't mean that you're automatically liberated from them. You may encounter new twists and turns of each of these illusions as you move through this book, so be sure to give yourself a refresher whenever you need a boost.

The same thinking applies to cultivating your still point. If the processes listed in chapter 5 are pushed to the far corners of your life and dusted off only during the occasional workshop or in a crisis, you won't reap their rewards. Choose one a week and give it some daily attention.

You are developing the capacity for a new relationship with movement. This requires some patience and practice. Here's how to know when you're tapping into your fitness instinct.

You'll start acting younger. Reawakening your fitness instinct triggers a playful mental attitude. You'll be willing to have fun with new ideas, stand apart from the orthodox, and explore and acquire new skills. Dr. David Weeks, a clinical neuropsychologist at the Royal Edinburgh Hospital in Scotland, and Jamie James, authors of *Secrets of the Superyoung*, believe that people who are younger than their biological ages don't censor themselves or expect others to do so. Highly adaptable, these age-resistant characters tend to be eccentric, giving themselves permission to engage in behavior that others might view as odd. The superyoung, according to Dr. Weeks, exercise regularly and enjoy a robust sex life.

You'll nourish your instinct to move. You'll start taking time to do the things that you know nourish and sustain your seventh sense, the instinct to move. The impulses to move are triggered by the deepest reverberations or vibrations in your body, as explained by the prana of Indian traditions and qi in the East. You can learn to sense this instinct and fan the glowing embers into a roaring blaze.

You'll connect with kindred movers. There is a philosophy in western Kenya that getting well and staying well is a tribal responsibility. *Harambee* is the Kiswahili word for unity that implies that no one is sick alone; everyone helps until the person gets well. While in Kenya, American medical student Shetal Shah discovered how harambee merges medicine with caring and culture and inspires families to learn how to give injections and take food to the hospital patient twice a day. A practice that first struck him as inefficient and perhaps unhygienic quickly taught him to relax in the face of communal wellness. Once you're fully in touch with holistic fitness, you move beyond an integration of mind, body, and spirit on a personal level and connect with the greater community, bio-region, and planet. You're only as well as your community.

7

Move to Your Internal Clock

Imagine being so in touch with your body's natural rhythms that the urge to move becomes irrepressible. You respond to an hour-by-hour demand by your internal time clock for moves that either energize, soothe, stabilize, or strengthen.

Welcome to *biorhythmic movement*, a complicated-sounding term that simply describes movement that caters to your biology and environment. Biorhythmic movement is the way you would naturally move, sense, breathe, and touch if you were freed from technological labor savers, body shame, and learned inhibitions.

This movement is governed mainly by circadian rhythms, the innate timekeepers for normal fluctuations in blood pressure, heart rate and rhythm, sleep and wakefulness, energy surges and dips, appetite, sexual responsiveness, mood, and alertness. As the day progresses, the shift from light to darkness influences your pineal gland, which triggers the production of various body chemicals. Like a million tiny scouts, they all seem bent on a mission to adjust your mood, energy level, appetite, and focus.

As you get in touch with this shifting, self-generating impulse to move, you learn to harness its energy based on the time of day. What I'm describing may seem impossible to sense right now, but in time and with practice, you will be able to do so.

All of the biorhythmic movements suggested throughout this chapter will bring you the benefits of better strength, endurance, and flexibility; enhanced energy; sustained calorie burn; and uplifted mood. I'll first explain which movements work best at which times of the day, then I'll explain how to match these moves to your movement personality.

DAWN: THE HEAD-TO-TOE KICKSTART

Morning requires moves that help you wake up and ready yourself for the day. Ideally, the best exercises stretch your spine, lubricate your joints, and stimulate circulation and energy. If you've learned qigong, tai chi, jin shin, yoga, or any martial arts, this is the best time of day for such disciplines. Other simple moves such as swinging a bat or golf club, using a hula hoop, jumping rope, or hopping on a trampoline also are great morning exercises.

This 20-minute Head-to-Toe Kickstart program is a blend of yoga, calisthenics, and qigong. The choreographed "flow" of moves seems to function as an ignition switch. What a kickstart does for a motorcycle, this does for your body. I predict that you will grow to love this dawn-inspired flow.

Do the routine in your bare feet on a cushioned mat or nonslip carpet. Pause in each of the strengthening postures for a few breaths, then move on to the next, paying attention to moving with fluidity and ease. Practice this at least once in the morning before eating. You can also do it at midday to reinvigorate yourself.

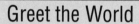

Greet the World

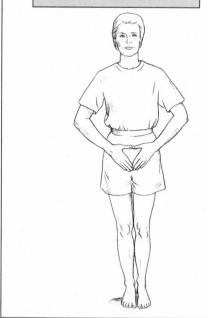

With your feet together, stand relaxed with your hands in a triangle position over your lower abdomen and your fingertips pointing down to the Earth. The triangle should outline your *tan tien*, a noted energy center approximately three finger-widths below your navel. Drop your shoulders as you breathe naturally and easily. Imagine a connection from the crown of your head to the sky and from the soles of your feet to the Earth's core. Greet your higher self or your source and give thanks. Breathe in the universal qi. Breathe out your intention for the day.

Hang

Bend your torso forward from the hips, exhaling as you let the weight of your head, arms, and upper body surrender to the pull of gravity. When you're starting out, keep your knees bent, and bend forward only as far as is comfortable. Eventually, as you gain flexibility, try to straighten your legs (you'll notice a mild stretch along your hamstrings). While you are in this pose, ask each part of you to relax so you grow heavy and warm. Focus on bending at your hip joints, not your midback. Imagine elongating your spine, opening up spaces between your vertebrae for stiffness to escape.

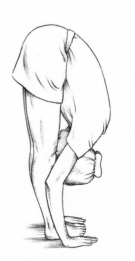

Downward Dog

Walk your hands forward while you adjust your feet to comfortably support this inverted V position. The flow of energy or prana is upward, from your hands through your shoulders and up your back to the end of your tailbone. Your head should hang loosely. Eventually, you will be able to bring your hands closer together, building strength in your shoulders. Energy is drawn from your strong, straight legs and from your heels pressing into the floor.

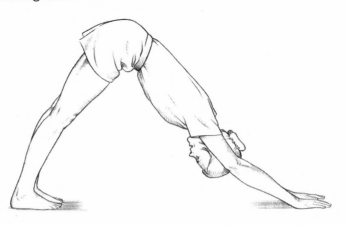

Plank

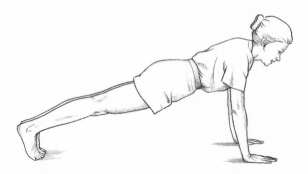

Come out of the dog by lowering your hips and moving your body forward, with your shoulders directly over your wrists. You should be balanced on your toes with your feet hip-width apart. Keep your abdominal muscles firm and your shoulders relaxed. Draw strength from the straight path that exists from the top of your head, through your shoulders and back, along your tailbone, down your legs, and to your toes.

Breathe into each joint that may feel pressure or congestion, such as your wrists or shoulders. Don't overfatigue any area; you're going to require a reservoir of strength to perform the next move.

Lowering Plank

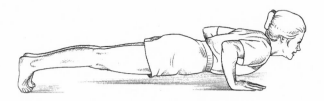

As you exhale, bend your elbows close to your sides and slowly lower your body in a straight line toward the floor. Don't worry if you can't do this move right away; it requires strength and may take several weeks or months to accomplish. You will be amazed at how quickly the backs of your arms become taut. In the beginning, you may lower your knees first to make the exercise easier.

Cobra

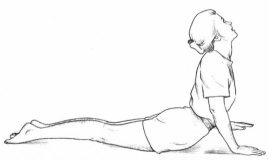

This time-honored posture opens your chest, elongates your abdominal cavity, builds strength, and stimulates energy. Lie flat on the floor with your legs outstretched, then inhale as you use your lower back muscles to lift your chest off the floor. Use your arms only for balance, not to push yourself higher. Keep your elbows pressed into the sides of your body. Let your eyeballs roll up and your mouth open slightly, and place the tip of your tongue on your upper palate.

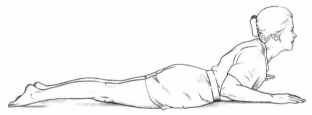

If you have lower back problems, modify the pose by lifting only the front of your chest and keeping your arms on the floor.

Surrender Stretch

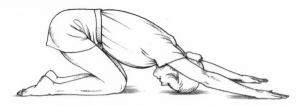

Let your forehead rest on the floor while you kneel back with your buttocks as close to your feet as possible. Keep your arms outstretched in front of you. This pose will stretch and relax your back.

Cat Stretch

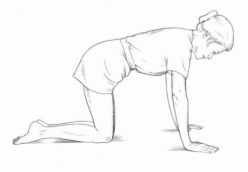

This sequence of strengthening and flexibility moves for the back will also build strength in your arms and shoulders. Begin on your hands and knees, with your fingers spread. Keep your spine neutral, neither tucking your hips under nor arching your back. Keep your head aligned with your spine so that your gaze is downward. Don't hunch your shoulders; move them away from your neck.

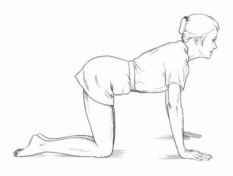

As you inhale, lift your chin and look up, allowing your back to sag as if a heavy saddle were being placed on it.

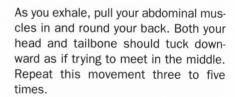

As you exhale, pull your abdominal muscles in and round your back. Both your head and tailbone should tuck downward as if trying to meet in the middle. Repeat this movement three to five times.

Once you have the basic body mechanics figured out, work on refining your breathing. Inhale and hold your breath while maintaining the arched spine. Release it after a few seconds and exhale slowly, drawing your navel in and bringing your head and tailbone down. Hold this position and breathe in and out a few times. Make sure that your face and neck muscles are not tense and your shoulders are down. As you inhale, return to the neutral spine position.

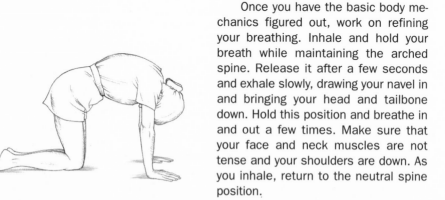

Pushup

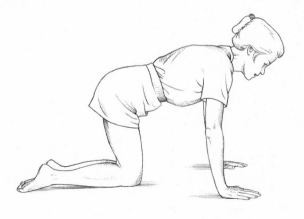

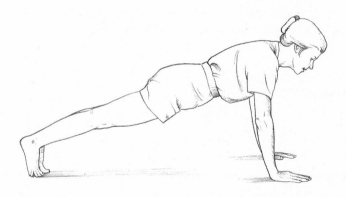

Pushups work your chest, upper arms, upper back, and shoulders. Beginners should keep their knees on the floor. Those with stronger upper bodies can advance to full pushups.

Keeping your elbows straight, place your hands on the floor slightly more than shoulder-width apart. Inhale as you bend your elbows and lower your chest toward the floor, then exhale as you push yourself up. Keep your abdominal muscles contracted for added support. At first, aim for a set of eight, but do as many as you comfortably can. Increase to two or three sets over time. Slow, controlled movements performed correctly will get you better results than dozens done the wrong way.

Lunge

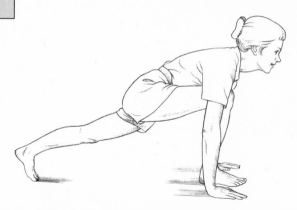

Place both hands on the floor and position your right foot between them, directly under your knee and shoulder. Inhale as you extend your left leg behind you, with the ball of your foot on the floor. Try to keep your leg extended as much as possible, but if you are uncomfortable, you can bend your left knee and rest it on the floor. Keep your chest up and your head aligned with your spine. This classic lunge will not only stretch your hip flexors (the very overworked muscles in the front of the groin) but will also increase strength throughout your extended leg.

Straight-Leg Stretch

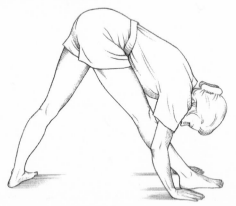

Keep your feet in the same position as for the previous exercise, then move your torso back and straighten your right leg completely. You should be leaning over your right leg with your hands flat on the floor.

Praising Warrior

Bend your right knee as you raise both arms into an overhead stretch. Your legs should be wide, with your right knee directly over your foot and your toes pointing forward. Your left foot should be angled slightly outward. Reach upward through your fingertips, keeping your shoulder blades down and back and pushing your chest forward. If you're a beginner, you can extend your arms in front of you until your balance improves.

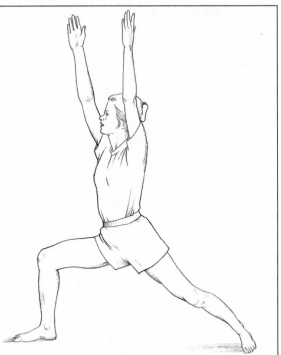

Warrior

With your legs in the same position as for the previous exercise, stretch your right arm to the front and your left to the rear. This is the classic warrior pose.

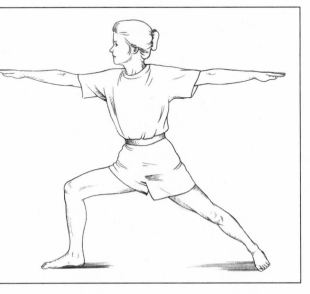

Half-Moon

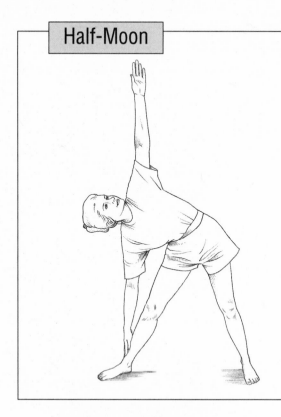

Straighten your right leg and raise your torso slightly. Exhale and shift your hips toward your left leg while you reach as far to the right as you can. Slowly lean your torso over your right leg, lowering it with control to the point of greatest stretch. The goal is to place your right hand on your right ankle, but if you can only reach your leg, that's fine—you will still get the benefit of the stretch. As you bend, stretch your left arm up, directly over your shoulder. Breathe easily, then inhale as you come out of the pose by bending your right leg slightly to reduce strain on your knees.

Wide-Leg Stretch

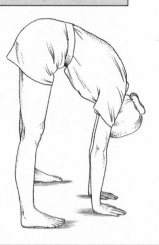

Pivot your feet so that you're standing with your legs widely spread. Lean forward from your hips, letting your arms and head hang down. You should feel a stretch along the insides of your legs. Next, come up slowly, placing your hands on your legs to help support your weight if necessary. Turn your left foot to the left and angle your right foot slightly outward in preparation for the next pose.

Lunge

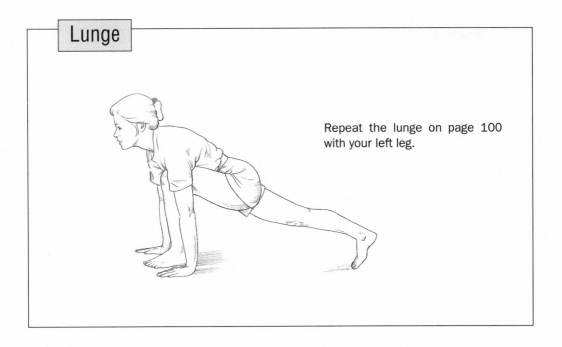

Repeat the lunge on page 100 with your left leg.

Straight-Leg Stretch

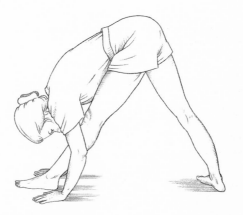

Repeat the stretch on page 100 to the left side by raising your hips and keeping your legs as straight as possible.

Praising Warrior

Repeat the pose on page 101 on your left side by bending your left knee as you raise your arms overhead.

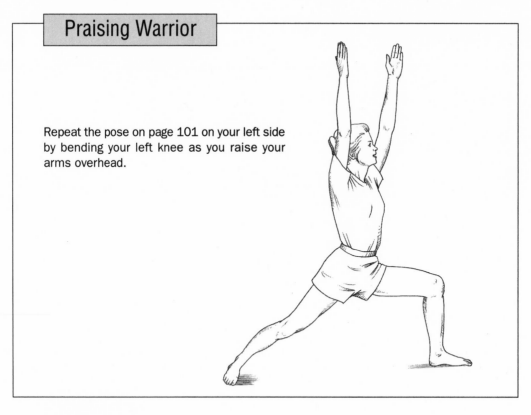

Warrior

Lower your arms into the shoulder-level extension, with one forward and one back. Repeat the full warrior pose on page 101, this time on your left side.

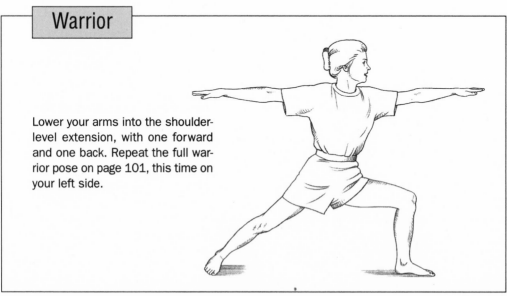

Half-Moon

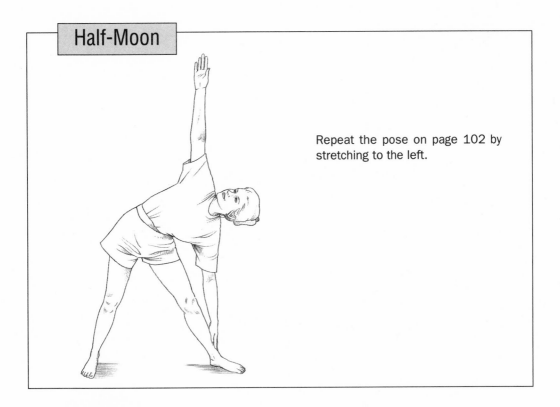

Repeat the pose on page 102 by stretching to the left.

Squat

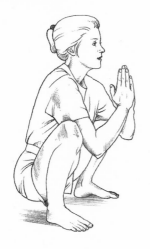

Come out of the half moon by lowering your arms to the floor and lowering your hips to support this squat. You may have to widen or narrow the position of your feet slightly to help yourself ease into the pose. Put your hands in a prayer position and press your upper arms or elbows into your knees for balance.

This is not an easy posture for most Westerners, but the full yoga squat is practiced by people in all native cultures and continued into advanced age. It offers benefits for the lower back and pelvic area. You can accomplish this pose slowly, with patience and much practice. Do not place your weight over your knees as in a deep knee bend; your weight should be centered in the pelvis. Do not try this position if you have problems with your knees.

Kneel

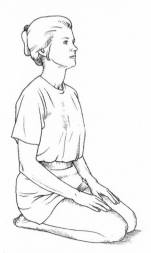

Recover from the squat by sitting with your buttocks on the backs of your lower legs. Acknowledge the openness you feel throughout your chest, hips, back, and joints. As you gain flexibility, try leaning back for an abdominal stretch by lifting your chest upward, arching backward, and supporting yourself with your hands behind you.

Butterfly

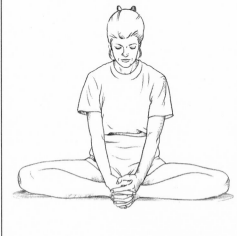

Supporting your weight with your hands, swing your legs around so that you are sitting with your knees bent and the soles of your feet touching. Fold your hands around your feet. The closer to the floor you can get your thighs, the more flexibility you are achieving in your hips. You can remain in this relaxed pose for up to three minutes. If you would like an added challenge, try to bend your torso so that your head approaches or touches each knee in turn. Then extend your legs in front of you.

V-Sit

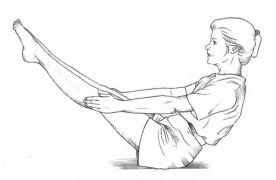

This challenging pose begins with you lying on your back, arms at your side. Take some deep breaths. When you're ready, slowly roll your upper back off the floor while bending your knees. Once you find a balanced position on your tailbone, attempt to straighten your legs. Hold this V position as long as you can, breathing normally as you do so, then slowly return to the starting position.

Full-Body Stretch

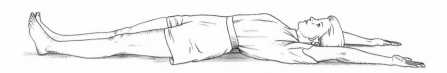

Lie on your back and stretch your arms behind your head for a relaxing, full-length stretch.

Cloud Walk

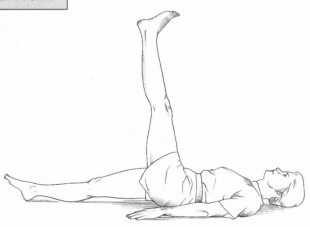

Do this move only if you have no lower back problems. Lie on your back with your arms at your sides and your legs outstretched. As you exhale, lift your left leg straight up in one strong movement. Then lift your upper torso as far as possible and try to touch your knee with your forehead. Return to the starting position and repeat with your right leg.

Knee to Chest

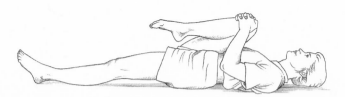

Still lying on your back, use your hands, either on your thigh or on your knee, to bring your right knee toward your chest. Try to keep your head on the floor, and breathe comfortably while you hold the position for at least 20 seconds to stretch your lower back, hips, and buttocks. Lower your leg, then raise your arms fully overhead and rest for a moment before repeating with your left knee.

Torso Stretch

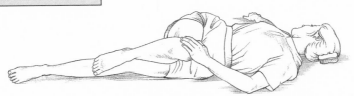

Lie on your back with your shoulders touching the floor and your arms outstretched to the sides. Keeping your left leg straight, bend your right leg so that your right foot is resting on your left knee. Turn your head to the right and use your left hand to gently push your right knee toward the floor. You will feel the stretch along your back and up your neck. Hold for a few breaths, then switch legs to stretch the other side.

Abdominal Curl

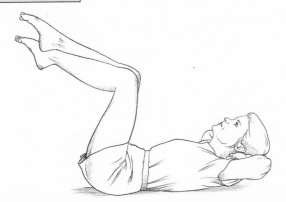

These are still the best overall means for strengthening your abdomen and thereby supporting your back. Lie on your back with your knees bent and your feet on the floor. Tuck your hips into a slight pelvic tilt so that your lower back is close to the floor, then raise your legs and cross one ankle over the other. Support the back of your head lightly with your fingertips. Your elbows should be extended to the sides, not close to your head. Keep your neck in good alignment with your spine; don't tuck your chin toward your chest. With a slow, controlled movement, lift your torso straight up until your shoulder blades clear the floor.

Exhale with each lift and pause slightly at the height of the contraction for an added challenge. Think of pulling your navel to the floor with each lift. Begin with eight lifts and work up to two sets. If you perform them correctly, there is no need to do an astronomical number of curls.

Oblique Curl

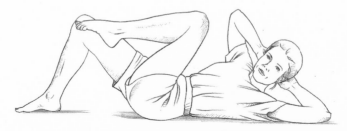

These are the best exercises to trim and tighten the muscles responsible for your waistline. Start in the same position as for the previous exercise, then raise your left leg. Lift your torso and rotate it diagonally, bringing the right side of your rib cage toward your left knee. Remember to keep your elbows out, and don't tuck your chin. Let your muscles do the work, not the momentum of swinging your body. Begin with eight on each side and advance to two or three more sets of eight.

Rest and Stretch

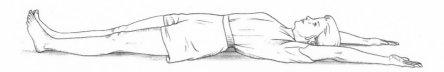

Do a full-body stretch as on page 107. Feel the work of the previous sequence. Release any tension that you may feel in your neck and shoulders, and feel yourself sinking and melting into the floor. Try a minute or two of deep breathing until you feel recharged.

Last Stretch

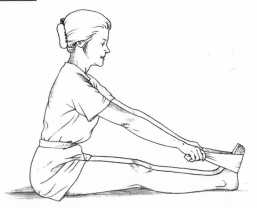

Give this last stretch in the sequence your best effort. Sit up and lean forward from the waist over your extended legs to get a full back, hip, upper leg, and hamstring stretch. Place a towel or exercise band around your feet and draw back gently, creating a pull on both legs.

Reflection

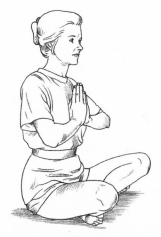

Seated in whatever position is most comfortable, move your hands out wide to the sides, then overhead, and finally down, imagining the energy flowing throughout your body and filling your heart. Let your hands come to rest at your chest. Enjoy a quiet moment of deep appreciation for your life.

DAYTIME: MOVEMENTS TO RE-ENERGIZE

Late morning and early afternoon require moves that stimulate your awareness, flood your brain with oxygen, boost your circulation, recharge your energy and enthusiasm, alleviate tension, and rid you of stress. Here are nine great ones.

Dance, dance, dance. Dancing is one of the most energizing activities you can do—and it's fun. If you have time during the day, take a one-hour break for a class in Middle Eastern dancing, better known as belly dancing. You can learn how to articulate your pelvis to the front and back, from side to side, and in figure eights—moves that strengthen your abdominal, oblique, lower back, and leg muscles.

Or, if you have just a few minutes, imitate a Latin salsa rhythm or let loose with your own jazz interpretation. If you have a partner, any swing dance can also be a great energizer.

Do the qigong twist. Standing with your legs hip-width apart and your knees slightly bent, rotate your pelvis fully from side to side without moving your feet. Let your arms fly until they stop themselves on your torso and swing back again.

Find a driving range. As you hit that bucket of golf balls, the movement you use is a very modified, Western version of a qigong twist.

Do your own thing. Improvisation can be applied to any number of expressive forms—dance, musical performance, poetry, comedy, or dramatic interpretation. The common element is that you make it up as you go, which can be extremely energizing because you must get in touch with intuition in order to be guided to your next gesture or sound.

Go to a pet-training class. Working closely with animals allows you to access intuition and eliminate stress. In order to communicate with animals, you have to join them in their agenda-free, instinctive world.

Take a walk. The ideal exercise, walking improves endurance, burns fat, prevents osteoporosis, cuts the risk of chronic disease, and elevates your mood. Brisk walks can be especially energizing during the day. Slower strolls can be meditative and soothing. Start with 10- to 20-minute walks and build up to 45 minutes over several weeks. Pick up your pace as you build muscle strength in your calves.

You can transform your gait into a smooth, effortless glide by breathing rhythmically and moving from your center. Elongate your body while you walk, lifting from your lower trunk and strengthening your crucial and often neglected postural muscles.

Try an aerobic lunch. If you can squeeze in a lunchtime aerobics class, you can get a second wind of energy and enthusiasm for the rest of the day. A well-designed class will take you through a safe warmup, sustain a workout that will build endurance and burn fat, and stretch major muscle groups at the conclusion.

Take a 10-minute run. What good is a very brief run? You'd be amazed. These 10-minute bursts are great because they're too short for you to work up a sweat (and therefore don't require an after-run shower) but are just long enough to lift your mood and provide a nice energy jolt. There are some guidelines, however.

- Wear comfortable, supportive shoes. While I did say earlier that shoes aren't necessary for many exercises, running is different. You need lots of good cushioning to do a quick run, because your body is not necessarily warmed up to the challenge.
- Keep it slow and steady. Aim for a pace that allows you to keep up a conversation. You shouldn't be at all breathless. Start slowly and build endurance over several weeks.
- Concentrate on time, not intensity. Think of what you're replacing with this 10-minute jog. Instead of seeking out coffee or sweets on a midday work break, you're actually burning about 100 calories.

Do a moveable treat. As mentioned in chapter 6, these exercises allow you to become playful and energetic. Some great daytime treats include nature

---

IN DEFENSE OF REST

People are invariably told to "squeeze in their workouts" on their 15-minute breaks, as if there were no value in resting at midday from an already overactive schedule. The resting state is actually extremely active. Repair and healing of cells and tissues and proper functioning of the immune system depend on prolonged states of rest.

Don't knock napping. Three-quarters of the world can't be wrong about it. When you need one, take a 10- or 15-minute power nap—and do it guiltlessly.

hikes, "getting down" to rock 'n' roll music, rock climbing, and city sight-seeing walks.

DUSK: MOVEMENTS TO SOOTHE, STABILIZE AND STRENGTHEN

Nighttime calls for moves that blast away stress, soothe anxiety and tension, and help your body unwind and regain equilibrium. It is also the best time to build strength. Here are some ways to achieve those goals.

➤ Soothing Movements

At the end of a long day, we all deserve to unwind. Try these gentle moves to pamper yourself.

Do the bear hug. With your knees slightly bent, let your torso fall forward slightly while stretching your arms across the front of your body and around toward your back, giving yourself a huge bear hug. Lower your head and breathe easily.

Come out of the bear hug with one slow, continuous opening of your arms. First open your arms straight out to the sides, then reach behind your back, attempting to bring your arms together behind you. Lift your head and open your chest. Flex your wrists to feel a stretch along your forearms. Bring your arms to the front very slowly, then repeat the bear hug. Do these movements three times.

Go swimming. A swim in warm water can be a blissful end to a busy day.

Stretch out. To reverse the forward crunch of working over a desk or computer, try rolling your shoulders backward. Next, bend forward from the waist to stretch your lower back and legs. Stand up and mimic the breast stroke, with just a small modification: Lead the motion with your thumbs. Next, mimic the backstroke with your little finger in the lead.

Stretch your head and shoulders. I call the area formed by your neck, shoulders, and midback the toxic dump of worries: It's where they seem to lodge forever, turning flesh into armor. Clean out the dump a few times a day (and especially before bed) with this move, a modified head roll.

First, stretch your neck forward, then to one side, with your ear toward your shoulder. Next, lift your chin straight up (don't roll your head too far back), then stretch toward the other shoulder before returning to center. With each quadrant, make sure that you feel a good stretch along your neck to your shoulder or to the midpoint between your shoulder blades. Assist the stretch by actively dropping your shoulders downward.

Lie on a tennis ball. Physical therapists created this easy way to reach the knots of stress and tension in lower-back muscles. Put a tennis ball in a small plastic bag. Lie on your back on the floor, place the ball at the base of your back, and gently roll around for a few minutes. Then reposition the ball so that you can roll it around the outline of your shoulder blades.

Shake off old qi. By the end of the day, qi, or your body's energy, grows stale and worn. It's time to create room for healing energy to restore and replenish you during the night. Start by rocking your torso, then let the shaking spread down your arms and legs and reach to your fingertips and feet. Work up to a vigorous shake, breathing deeply and imagining that you're ridding

GET IN TOUCH WITH THE PLANET

Time is not the only factor that affects how you move each day; place does as well. A myriad of ways exist for us to connect with the places we call home. From knowing where our garbage is processed to predicting the sunset, we grow closer to taking good care of ourselves when we engender a more intimate, accountable, and aware relationship with the natural world we live in.

If we open ourselves to the possibility of a place to shape us, we enter into an inexhaustible relationship of give-and-take. Together, you and your place feed each other. In what physical ways can you participate more fully with your environment? First, there are the obvious yardwork, shoveling, gardening, and home repair projects. Then there are community trail repair and stream cleaning. My kids and I love to liberate streams after the heavy rains in Northern California. It's a full day of exhausting work in which all of your muscles join in the scraping, lifting, hauling, balancing, and tossing. In the end, you sit on a boulder and watch the stagnant ponds transform into clear, clean, running rapids.

You may be thinking, "Fine. I'd love to be challenged by the great outdoors all day, but I have a job and responsibilities that keep me tied to my present situation. I can't overhaul my life." Realize that I'm not asking you to make any major changes; I'm just asking you to consider small, incremental ones that you can slowly initiate. Start by adding a few outdoor, natural endeavors once a week. Schedule one weekend a month in a natural setting. Eventually, you'll find ways to include natural activities every day, because you'll be inspired by your surroundings and you'll sense more possibilities.

yourself of old, stale energy. Shake off the hassles, the unfinished business, the nagging voices, and the frustrations of the day. Keep it up for at least one minute. When you're finished, stand with your eyes closed and your palms facing up.

Try de-stressing soothers. These stress-reducing strategies are more fully explained in chapter 6. Basically, any of the following will provide a nice, soothing end to the day: meditation, visualization, yoga poses, massage, and drumming.

➤ Strengthening Movements

Doing 20 quick pushups before hitting the sack is actually a good idea. It diverts blood to the working muscles and away from the brain, allowing your

---

THE SECRETS OF BODY WISDOM

Members of some of the world's cultures show the beauty of biorhythmic movement at its best. These people from Thailand, the Sudan, and Peru move in alignment with the hormonal shifts within their bodies, the hours of the day, and the seasons of the year. We have a lot to learn from people who live in some of the poorest nations of the world. While they may lack fancy gadgets, cars, and houses, they have a secret gift: body wisdom. Here are some of those secrets.

Eat qi for breakfast. Instead of eating first thing in the morning, try filling yourself with qi, the energy that radiates from the natural world. The Thai mountain people taught me to stand barefoot on the Earth in the early morning, breathe deeply, and draw the abundant energy into my body. As I exhaled, I emptied out the old, stale energy.

Discover muscle inefficiency. In our clamor to create efficient timesaving and labor-saving systems and devices, we burn 500 to 800 fewer calories a day. Not the Thai mountain dwellers. When they plant, they squat rather than sitting. They use five pots when they cook rather than one. Every event entails a flurry of movement. Learn from them by making every simple task as difficult as you can. Instead of moving two muscle groups to accomplish something, involve your whole body. You can double your calorie output in a single day.

Burn fat all day long. The Nepalese showed me that it is possible to move while you're resting. In native cultures, people work harder but in shorter spurts. Rest and mental chatterbox to wind down for a good night's rest. Challenging your muscles before you sleep will put your body in a glycogen-needy state by early morning. Then, if you do any aerobic activity such as walking or cycling, you will tap into more fat reserves than usual. Here are some choices of exercises to try before bed, but don't pick more than two. If you exhaust yourself, you'll actually find it tough to sleep.

- 12 high knee lifts (Jogging slowly in place.)
- 12 jumping jacks
- 12 burpees (Remember these from grade school? Stand, drop your hands to the floor, kick your legs out behind you, bring them back, and then stand.)

play are interwoven with more frequency, making rest periods not simply times for collapse but opportunities for play, dance, and easy movement.

Dance the day away. The Nubians of northern Sudan dance while they work, while they rest, and while they converse with friends and family. I fell in love with their call-response mode of singing and dancing. Nubian movement looks like the genetic mother of jazz and hip-hop. Dance to some African drumming music and let your feet, hands, head, and spine trace different rhythms. You'll blow the carbon off your "engine."

The small drum that I carried with me on my global travels proved to be my smartest satchel. A cross-cultural ice-breaker, the drum is a universal communication tool. Pound out a catchy rhythm, and soon hips are swaying, smiles are beaming, and, in five minutes, you have the makings of a wild rumpus. Dance with wild abandon at least once a day. Dance your tears, joys, fears, and prayers. Stash your "Top 40" for a while and pick up some African drum music. Let the music move you.

Climb hills; carry water. Lifting and carrying heavy objects has disappeared from our daily routines. Instead we push grocery carts, drag luggage with wheels, and use conveyor belts for everything. Take note of how many times you make it easier on yourself by avoiding a long carry or a heavy lift. Native people carry heavy objects by supporting them on their upper backs and heads, not by toting them in front of their bellies. This requires a lifetime of practice, starting with lighter weights and building up slowly.

- 12 lunges (See page 100; do 6 with each leg.)
- 12 squats (See page 1056.)
- 12 step-ups (These are as easy as they sound. Step up onto a six-inch-high stool, step, or sturdy box, making sure both feet are planted solidly, then step down. Repeat, leading with the same leg, then switch legs.)
- 12 chair dips (Sit on the very edge of a stable chair with your palms on the seat next to your buttocks. Slide your buttocks off the chair and support your weight with your hands. Lower yourself toward the floor as you bend your elbows behind you, then return to the starting position.)
- 12 V-sits (See page 107.)
- 12 abdominal curls (See page 109.)
- 12 pushups (See page 99.)
- 12-count rest in surrender stretch (See page 97.)

➤ Stabilizing Movements

Like strengthening, the following stabilizing moves will help you unwind before bed while strengthening your back. They are borrowed from Pilates, which uses carefully controlled, precise movements to improve strength and flexibility without bulking up your body. Do the moves on a mat or carpeted floor.

Back Lift

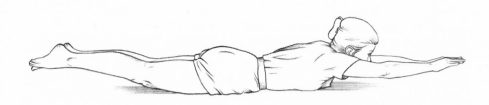

Lying face down, exhale and pull your abs in toward your spine. Extend your arms straight out above your head, straighten your legs, squeeze your buttocks, and lift your arms and legs slightly. Breathe easily and then relax. For an added challenge, lift your head and shoulders as well.

All-Fours Stretch

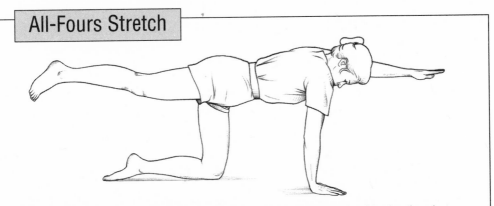

Kneel on all fours, then extend your left arm in front of you at shoulder level and your right leg behind you at hip level. Push out through your longest finger and your heel. Imagine that you're extending a line of energy that can touch the walls. Breathe easily and balance for at least 20 seconds before switching sides.

Leg Sweep

Stand tall, with your rib cage lifted, your shoulders relaxed, and your arms slightly out from your sides for balance. Sweep your right leg in front of your left, balancing on your left foot (you will wobble a little in the beginning). Hold for as long as you can, then switch sides.

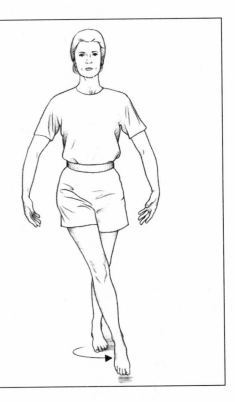

Stork

Stand tall and move your left foot as high as you can against the inside of your right leg. To increase the balancing challenge, raise your arms overhead in a prayer position. Hold for as long as you can, then switch legs.

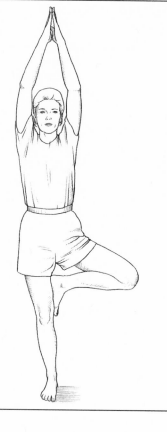

Pelvic Circles

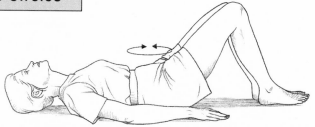

Lie on your back with your knees bent and your arms at your sides. Keeping the small of your back on the floor, concentrate on moving your pelvis in small circles, first clockwise, then counterclockwise. You'll feel the massage in your lower back. Breathe easily and move as slowly as possible.

Flexor Stretch

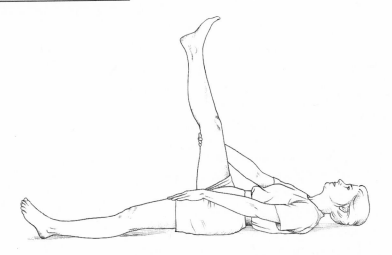

Lie on your back with both legs straight out on the floor, then raise your right leg perpendicular to the floor. Place your right hand on the back of your thigh, right above the knee, to support it. This will give you a mild hamstring stretch in the raised leg, but to stretch the hip flexors, you need to concentrate on your left leg, which is flat on the floor. If raising your right leg makes your left thigh pop off the floor, you have tight hip flexors that need stretching. Take your free hand and gently push at the groin to coax your thigh down to the floor. Repeat with your left leg. Since hip flexors are notoriously tight, they need to be stretched regularly.

TIME AND YOUR MOVEMENT TYPE

Now that you know which moves generally work best at which times of day, you are ready to customize that information to your personality.

Why the need to customize? It's because circadian energy patterns vary considerably among the four movement types. Racers thrive in the early morning, for example, while Trekkers can't get energized until late morning. The following menus of biorhythmic movements are designed to round out your energies so you burn calories more efficiently. Moreover, they will make you feel appropriately energized, active, and rested throughout your waking hours.

Note that most of these movements take just a few minutes. By "dancing," I mean that you should put on one great song and let go for just three minutes, then return to your business. When I say "brisk walking," I mean just five minutes.

Of course, these aren't your only movement options. Chapter 9 goes into more detail about how to achieve the right balance among aerobic, strengthening, and stretching movements throughout the day. My hope here is to give you a template for doing a few minutes of exertion every waking hour, in a sequence that best suits your body's unique rhythms. The goal is to make it a lifelong habit. It takes practice, but it's worth it. The health benefits are immeasurable. It is the natural way for humans to move; people in native cultures throughout the world thrive by spreading their movements throughout the day rather than going for a single spurt of high-intensity exertion at a gym.

→ Racer

Morning is usually your most energetic time, with your stamina falling straight through to a lethargic dip from 11:00 A.M. to 1:00 P.M. You usually get a second wind in midafternoon, but it is brief, and you soon crash. A third energetic wave takes place in the late evening. Racers are true night owls. In Ayurvedic terms, they have an aggravated pitta, which gives them a fiery drive, and they should avoid exercising when it's very hot.

To even out these surges and dips, you'll need to capitalize on your natural high energy in the morning while extending your fiery vital energies into late afternoon. The following moves at the times indicated will increase your capacity for sustaining energy and offer a safe, easy framework for building power and strength in the evening.

7:00 A.M.: Kickstart moves (three to five from the program on page 94).

8:00 A.M.: Kickstart moves (three to five).

9:00 A.M.: Moveable treat, such as boogying to your favorite song.

10:00 A.M.: Energizing visualization.

11:00 A.M.: Dancing.

Noon: Brisk walking.

1:00 P.M.: De-stressing soother, such as meditation or yoga.

2:00 P.M.: Breathing exercise.

3:00 P.M.: Quick hopping.

4:00 P.M.: Quick burst of speedwalking.

5:00 P.M.: Deep breathing.

6:00 P.M.: Brisk walking or dancing.

7:00 P.M.: Strengthening movements (three or four from page 116).

8:00 P.M.: Stabilizing movements (two from page 118).

9:00 P.M.: Old qi shake-off (see page 115).

⊚ Stroller

Quiet morning hours usually give rise to a strong peak of energy from 10:00 A.M. to 2:00 P.M., when you are most productive. You are also able to mount a secondary energetic wave from around 4:00 to 7:00 P.M., but by 9:00 P.M., you're practically brain-dead.

Strollers need to focus and strengthen their energy for metered output throughout the day. The following routine will stimulate vitality and quickness, burn calories, and build on opportunities for play and recreation.

7:00 A.M.: Brisk walking or running.

8:00 A.M.: Morning chores, performed with big muscle moves.

9:00 A.M.: Energizing visualization.

10:00 A.M.: Light calisthenics.

11:00 A.M.: Dancing.

Noon: Brisk walking.

1:00 P.M.: Soothing movements (see page 114).

2:00 P.M.: Yoga breath-of-fire exercise: Begin with a forceful exhalation, triggered by pulling your abdominal muscles in suddenly. Follow with a passive inhalation, letting your muscles relax and allowing air to enter your lungs. Repeat this cycle of forceful-out, passive-in at an even pace of about one breath every three seconds, but not so fast that you hyperventilate. Do no more than 10 cycles in the beginning; after a few weeks, you can progress to 20. This ancient practice will oxygenate your blood, maximize the clearing of carbon dioxide and other wastes, exercise your diaphragm, massage your intestines, build a bioelectric charge that helps focus your attention, clear your mind, and ignite your energy.

3:00 P.M.: Quick hopping.

4:00 P.M.: Quick burst of speedwalking.

5:00 P.M.: Six-directional breathing exercise (see page 69).

6:00 P.M.: Brisk walking.

7:00 P.M.: Strengthening movements (three from page 116).

8:00 P.M.: Stabilizing movements (two from page 118).

9:00 P.M.: Old qi shake-off (see page 115).

✳ Dancer

Your major energy wave is long and well-sustained through midafternoon until 5:00 P.M. You have a fairly substantial energy peak in early morning from 6:00 to 9:00 A.M. Your dip occurs in the early evening from 7:00 to 10:00 P.M. Sometimes a nap at this time will trigger a restless night.

Dancers can enhance fluidity, balance, grace, posture, and poise with the following moves. This routine will also increase circulation and mental preparedness for the day, quicken creative energies, and prevent sluggishness, providing an outlet for a late-afternoon energy jolt.

7:00 A.M.: Walking meditation (see page 71).
8:00 A.M.: Energizing visualization.
9:00 A.M.: Head-to-Toe Kickstart (see page 94).
10:00 A.M.: Yoga breath-of-fire exercise (see page 124).
11:00 A.M.: Dancing.
Noon: Brisk walking.
1:00 P.M.: Five minutes of jumping rope.
2:00 P.M.: Simple deep breathing.
3:00 P.M.: Any recreational movements, such as walking, running, skating, or bicycling.
4:00 P.M.: Energy-generating movements, such as jumping rope or doing yoga.
5:00 P.M.: Uphill hike.
6:00 P.M.: Belly dancing or gardening.
7:00 P.M.: Soothing visualization.
8:00 P.M.: Stabilizing movements (two from page 118).
9:00 P.M.: Strengthening movements (two from page 116).
10:00 P.M.: Old qi shake-off (see page 115).

⌐⌐ Trekker

As an early riser, you experience a short spurt of energy from 5:00 to 7:00 A.M. but usually have to force yourself to stay alert from 11:00 A.M. to 2:00 P.M. This should be your siesta, since the dip is quite significant. Your energy is sustained fairly well in the afternoon, with the big peak coming during the late evening hours. Trekkers enjoy working late at night with no one to bother them.

This routine will slowly generate energy in the morning, awaken your sluggish system during early midday, and provide sustaining power late in the evening while still calming you for a good night's rest.

9:00 A.M.: Qigong twist (see page 112).
10:00 A.M.: Walking meditation (see page 71).
11:00 A.M.: Energizing visualization.
Noon: Head-to-Toe Kickstart (see page 94).
1:00 P.M.: Play or recreation break.
2:00 P.M.: Yoga breath-of-fire exercise (see page 124).
3:00 P.M.: Jumping rope.
4:00 P.M.: Quick, brisk walk.
5:00 P.M.: Nature hike.
6:00 P.M.: Building sand castles.
7:00 P.M.: Yoga.
8:00 P.M.: Stabilizing movements (two from page 118).
9:00 P.M.: Strengthening movements (two from page 116).
10:00 P.M.: Old qi shake-off (see page 115).
11:00 P.M.: Soothing visualization.

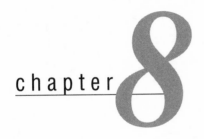

chapter 8

Explore Alternative Moves

You've probably already heard about alternative healing, which uses remedies such as herbs, acupuncture, and massage. These remedies reap lots of positive results, and recently, they have been earning more respect from Western medicine.

Well, I'm now going to bring you the exciting world of alternative fitness, a wide range of activities that run counter to just about everything the fitness industry stands for. These forms of fitness engage you from head to toe, from your subconscious inner world to your conscious outer state of being, from your spiritual crown to your earthly root chakras, or energy points. Alternative fitness moves are always engaging, sometimes challenging, and never exhausting. They work from the inside out. They are intuitive fitness at its best—fitness activities that you will love.

Alternative moves decrease stress and promote pleasure with the intention of attaining a different, deeper, more integrated, and holistic level of wellness and fitness. They are based on flow.

University of Chicago researcher Mihaly Csikszentmihalyi, Ph.D., has been studying the optimal experience of flow states for nearly three decades. He says that everyone experiences flow states from time to time, and he describes those states as periods of peak contentment, when a "state of concentration is so focused that it amounts to absolute absorption in an activity."

When you feel strong, alert, and unselfconscious, as if the control you are exerting is completely effortless, you've tapped into a flow state. Flow states help us achieve harmony and happiness, and luckily, they can be accessed regularly. Where does flow show up in your life? Try sports, sensual delights, work relationships, yoga, music, and solitude. Once you experience flow during movement, it will soon spill over into the rest of your life. Suddenly, you will find a heightened sense of consciousness and mastery over your life. Tasks become joyful, effortless, and stress-free. Is this too much to ask from a 30-minute excursion into alternative fitness? Maybe, but it's a good place to start.

WHY GO ALTERNATIVE?

Tightness. Pain. Stress. Tension. Conventional exercise powers through these sensations, working toward a specific goal of getting stronger, faster, and leaner. Alternative fitness uses such sensations to get to the underlying causes, explore the source of the tension, and work toward the release of the chronic holding pattern. In this way, you open yourself to more flexibility and movement options.

The difference here is echoed in medicine. Much of conventional medicine focuses on eliminating discomfort and symptoms through pharmaceuticals and other interventions, whereas alternative systems of healing, such as naturopathy, look at symptoms as informants, clues that lead to the underlying problem.

The following are some of my favorite alternative fitness paths because they provide practical techniques that most people can easily learn, along with interesting excursions for your mind, body, and spirit.

➤ Authentic Movement

People who don't enjoy dancing usually worry too much about what others will think. Yet, there is no wrong way to dance, as long as you move with the natural surges produced by your body. Authentic movement is a form of expressive-acts therapy based on the principles of pioneering psychiatrist Carl Jung. It teaches you to move naturally to the spontaneous flow that your body produces. What better way to tap into your fitness instinct?

Taking a class or workshop in authentic movement is an excellent way to learn how to really feel your body's intuitive movement while bypassing your

REAL-LIFE INSTINCTS

Diane, 28, laughed about her first experience in an authentic movement class. It was simply "too weird" for her. "The teacher kept saying, 'Move from your center,' as if I knew where the heck my center was . . . and also, 'Go where your body wants to go.' Ha! My body? How was I supposed to know? My mind wanted to head straight for the door. Maybe get something to eat—that's probably what my body wanted!"

I chuckled right along with her because I remembered how foreign and dispossessed I felt in my first experiential dance class. I was like an ugly duckling out of the pond, exposed for all my inexperience and lack of physical grace.

After years of sticking my toe back in the water, however, taking more classes in bodywork, dance, somatic education, and movement analysis, I've come to respect the language and the wisdom that support this rich and varied field—what bodyworker and author Mirka Knaster calls "body ways." We can embark on a coming-home journey in terms of residing in our bodies. It's slow and windy and replete with both joyful and poignant memories. Stay on the path. It's worth it.

brain's self-critical thoughts. Instead of using exercise as a way to avoid feeling, you can enhance the quality of your life through movement that engages your feelings. As you begin an authentic movement class, Nancy Minges, Restorative Fitness director at the Claremont Resort and Spa in Oakland, California, offers these questions.

- Can you allow yourself to feel the movements more deeply?
- Can you release the anticipation of movement?
- Can you move from your center and not from your head?
- Where is your body trying too hard or struggling?
- Where do you feel pockets of unnecessary tension?
- What is the story that your body is trying to tell you?

Authentic movement is properly done with a witness, who watches in a silent, nonjudgmental way. When you're finished moving, your friend describes what she saw. If you don't have or don't want someone to watch you, you can still try authentic movement. Warm up to it by simply moving in your own living room to some favorite music without lyrics. Try starting out on the floor with your eyes closed, and keep the movements small and contained. Tap in to what moves you instead of having your head direct your body.

For information on classes, contact the California Institute of Integral Studies, 1453 Mission Street, San Francisco, CA 94103.

➤ Climbing

This demanding sport is so popular that at first, you probably wouldn't think of it as alternative. I do, because of its total insistence on your mindful attention. Rock and wall climbing both bring life and death into the equation, no matter how many belays you have rigged. After you've climbed a wall, you'll realize how hard your mind was working and how few distracting thoughts crept into your head.

You can start safely by taking a beginner class at an indoor climbing gym, where the floors are padded, belays are plentiful, and the artificial rocks are a bit easier to navigate than the real, outdoor thing. Check with clubs in your area to see if they have climbing walls, and be sure to ask if their trainers are certified climbing instructors.

If you're in California, check out Vertical Hold in San Diego. In Boston, try the Ski and Sports Club. Both are wonderful climbing gyms.

➤ Continuum

This technique was developed by French dance innovator Emilie Conrad Da'oud, and its practitioners believe that movement is something we are rather than something we do. In many ways, it is the most psycho-emotionally therapeutic of all the alternative fitness techniques listed in this book.

Continuum teachers talk about connecting cellularly, viscerally, and neuromuscularly to the flow of life. A session with a certified teacher is unlike anything you've ever done. The technique centers around "micro movements" that are done at an excruciatingly slow pace. You will be amazed at the difficulty you may encounter. Just moving that slowly will pull up emotional content for you: old memories, buried anger, forgotten joys.

For more information on Continuum, write to 1629 18th Avenue, #7, Santa Monica, CA 90404, or look for Continuum teachers in your area.

▶ Dynamic Walking

At first glance, you'd think that Suki Munsell, Ph.D., is just teaching people to walk better, and in one sense, she is. As a movement expert, Dr. Munsell, founder of the Dynamic Health and Fitness Institute in Corte Madera, California, teaches you to retrain your hip flexors to release, lift your hips and trunk, and swing your legs, creating more glide and less impact. That's just the biomechanical side of her dynamic walking program, however. On a deeper level, she uses her 24 years as a registered movement therapist to help people, at every stage of life and with various illnesses and disabilities, recover a healthy body image.

For her doctoral research, Dr. Munsell studied how people could success-fully overcome disfigurement, birth defects, illness, and injury by simply and consistently imagining themselves moving in a positive way. The degree of con-sistency with the "imagined body" is the key to working positively with certain dynamic principles. As a somatic practitioner (see "Somatics" on page 141), Dr. Munsell also helps clients release blocked emotions and subpersonalities with dynamic walking. Just bringing awareness and a flow of energy into areas that were tightly held can bring an unexpected emotional outburst.

Respect for proper form and posture is, of course, another element of her program. If you don't get the base of your body in contact with the ground to support your upper body well, you send the pyschobiological message, "I don't have a leg to stand on," to the rest of yourself. As a result, you cause some tightening—called compensatory constriction—farther up your muscular frame that "affects your personality and your pathology," says Dr. Munsell.

Some 1,000 instructors have been certified in the dynamic walking method. For more information, call the Dynamic Health and Fitness Institute at (888) 852-6717, or send e-mail to dynamics@well.com.

▶ Eastern Power Classes

Kind of a potpourri of various martial arts disciplines, Eastern power can include everything from basic self-defense moves to a good measure of tai chi for grace and agility. Many classes blend Asian techniques for mastering bal-ance, coordination, power, and inner peace, and they may also help challenge your muscles in new ways.

You will find these classes taught predominantly in clubs in San Francisco

(continued on page 134)

MY THINKING ON CYCLING

It's fun, it's outdoors, it's healthy—is there anything negative to say about this increasingly popular pastime? Since so much variety exists within the sport of cycling, there's a style to suit every movement personality. From daily rides, quick jaunts to the store, regular club events, mountain trail rides, and races to long-distance touring, multiday rides, and BMX events, cycling has a lot of different faces!

What type of bike is right for you? The choices are essentially mountain, road, and hybrid. The only way you'll know what's right for you is to try them out. For the last 10 years, mountain bikes were the top sellers, but lately there's been a shift back to road bikes, according to Joshua Gallup of Bicycle Connection in Moraga, California. Let convenience, common sense, personal ability, and preference help guide your choice.

If you live in an area with easy access to dirt trails, you may want to consider an off-road bike to enjoy some nature excursions and get one of the best workouts on record. Borrow a friend's bike and test it on an easy trail before you decide, though. If you commit to a mountain bike and then find that you'd rather just be a street recreationalist, you'll be sorry that you're lugging those heavy tires around.

Is it possible for you to commute to work on your bike? If so, you have a ready-made way to stay fit and green the planet by improving air quality at the same time. As more cities respond to the increasing demands for safe cycling programs, we will see more designated bike lanes and bicycle awareness programs.

Some of the most imaginative vacations in the world are designed by cycle tour companies. On trips such as rides through the Colorado mountains (offered by Scenic Cycling Adventures; 800-413-8432) or tours of the United Kingdom and Europe, you'll meet fellow cyclists and enjoy the luxurious support of vans, lodging, campsites, meals, and rental bikes.

Even if you think that you'll never be more than a weekend-only, recreational cyclist, you'll still want to invest in a well-built, reliable bike in order to really enjoy the sport. You'll probably need to spend between $499 and $1,500. The higher-priced bikes are faster and lighter, and for $3,000, you can even get the new disc brakes. Well-known brands include Trek, Cannondale, and Fisher.

What about comfort? Incorrect bike fit is probably the number one cause of excessive fatigue and discomfort when cycling. A good bike shop will help you determine the right bike size for your legs, the right forward stretch for your torso, and the best arm and hand positions, based on your ability and the type of cycling you'll be doing. Don't aim for a riding position that you think looks racy if it causes you continuous strain.

Serious enthusiasts always encounter risks and injuries specific to their particular sport. For cycling, that means groin numbness, which can lead to serious problems for men. One way to avoid the problem is with a seat that features a gel pad in a cut-out portion of the seat under the groin. Wearing well-padded cycling shorts and using the correct riding position are also crucial for avoiding discomfort.

When it comes to training, avid cyclists will tell you to put in your hours on the road or the dirt—that there really is no substitute for the real activity. Cross-training can include weight lifting, inline skating, cross-country skiing, and running, which are all perfect for building strength in your lower body. And don't forget a dedicated program of weight training for your upper body, shoulders, and arms as well, since they'll undergo new challenges of sustained tension and endurance.

You could also take an indoor cycling class such as Spinning or Power Pacing to build your strength. Even if you're an experienced outdoor cyclist, these classes can be tough in the beginning, so be sure to work within your limits. You can control the pedaling resistance by turning a knob that tightens felt pads on the flywheel. Tightening the pads simulates the sensation of pedaling uphill. In a 45-minute class, you can practice sprints, jumps, and hill climbing. Your instructor will call out various moves while helping you visualize the terrain shifting, sometimes to music.

With all forms of cycling, be sure to stretch your calves, hamstrings, and quads after each session. Also, put your upper body through some stretches, including some dedicated flexibility moves for your wrists, forearms, and shoulders.

and Los Angeles, due to their proximity to the Pacific Rim. Recently, however, classes have been spilling over into most urban centers. Sometimes, they are taught under the classical names tai chi, tae kwon do, or aikido.

When these Asian techniques are thrown into the wild multicultural mix here in the United States, enterprising teachers merge concepts of various disciplines and blend them with their own dance or aerobic choreography. One innovative teacher, Carol Argo, has even taken her tai chi class to the water.

Such techniques may be a serious breach of a discipline's teaching in Asia, and some purists consider them abominations. I tend to think that this creative license tailors the moves to the style and consciousness of the new locale and its people.

➤ Emotional Fitness

Once a television actress, Elisa Lodge transformed her life after she studied with legends of body-oriented therapy such as Fritz Perls, Ida Rolf, and Moshe Feldenkrais. Today, she is masterful at helping people recognize and release old habits, limiting attitudes, and conformist postures that hold them back from true personal power and what she calls natural fitness.

Inspiring her students to regain spontaneity, ease, and playfulness in their quest for healthy, fit bodies, Lodge is one of the most popular workshop leaders at the Esalen Institute in Big Sur, California. With her partner James Wanless, she consults for corporations, wellness centers, and spas on Ageless Vitality and other transformative movement workshops. Breaking the boundaries of conventional training, Lodge employs her vast talents in theater, comedy, and vocal arts to teach others how to make breath, sound, and movement parts of natural fitness.

One of her gifts lies in helping people during major transitions. During stressful times of loss or separation, we have a tendency to neglect our bodies, which causes a loss of vigor and flexibility. When emotions are stuck, the body becomes rigid. As a neuromuscular retrainer, Lodge helps catalyze that emotion into a vast, unlimited power that can creatively shape and shift your body into a performing work of art. She showed me how during a transitional time in my life, and I'll always be grateful to her.

For information about national seminars, workshops and training sessions, write to Emotional Fitness, 26015 Dougherty Place, Carmel, CA 93923, or send e-mail to e-motion@webtv.net.

➤ The Flow

If you're a clumsy sort who never really knows where your arms or feet will land next, the flow is for you. This motion awareness system has you move with a water-filled polyurethane sleeve that looks something like a condom sized for a blue whale. Developed by martial arts master Victor Blome, the flow provides students with a biofeedback gauge. If your movements are jerky or your breathing is unsteady, the flow of water becomes choppy. Once you settle into a flow state, the water glides around you as if you were a peaceful shore.

To enjoy the flow, you slip your hands into the secure handles at each end of the two-pound device and direct it overhead, from side to side, behind you, through your legs, around you—there's no limit to the number of combinations. While you're getting a cardiovascular challenge, you're also getting an incredible upper-body workout, a moderate lower-body workout, and a soothing mental vacation. Flow addresses balance, coordination, flexibility, and agility, but most of all, it enables you to make new neuromuscular connections, freeing yourself from fixed and rigid patterns that limit your kinesthetic options. The flow is based in Austin, Texas. Look for classes like it near you.

➤ Hiking

There is really nothing alternative about hiking as an activity; it shows up on most lists of various recommended types of aerobic exercise. I'm referring, however, to a special kind of ecological hiking. If you've ever been on a trail, you've seen people who stride past at break-neck speed, with their eyes focused on the uneven ground as they move at a pace that would be better accomplished on a treadmill. Ecological hiking, on the other hand, means waking up to your surroundings, carrying a plastic bag, stopping to pick up litter, clearing a stream when needed, and basically noticing where you are and contemplating your fortunate inclusion in this grand web of life. The pace is secondary to the total experience.

Few activities in the world can rival the splendor of hiking through lush hills, up the summits of rocky peaks, along breathtaking waterfalls, or through peaceful valleys. I consider hiking the perfect exercise because it combines a physical challenge with a respite for your mind and emotions. Even if you take to the woods with a head full of worries, you'll soon be stepping with a lighter load, because time spent in nature gives you a new perspective that helps you put priorities back in order and uncover hidden solutions.

If you're fortunate enough to live near some areas with marked trails, your life could take on a higher quality if you hike for at least a few hours every week. Once you get used to your hiking excursions, you won't want to be without them.

Angeles Arrien, a cultural anthropologist and author, told me that she has to spend an "uncompromisable" hour a day outdoors, away from it all. Confirmed hikers and walkers treat themselves to special travel adventures once or twice a year.

You can plan these trips yourself by writing to the federal and state parks and preservation lands you wish to visit, or you can let some hiking pros do the planning for you. There are many hiking companies that provide expert guides, tested trails, and well-planned itineraries. You can experience the outdoors by day and be cozy in a country inn by night.

Clare and Kurt Grabher run New England Hiking Holidays, which, despite the name, offers guided hiking and walking holidays from New England to the Blue Ridge Mountains, throughout the Rockies and Sierras, and in Europe, Canada, and Hawaii. Call them at (800) 869-0949.

Another favorite is Jimmy LeSage's New Life Hiking Spa, which has been promoting hiking instead of pampering as a vacation alternative for two decades. If you want to recharge at this hiking hideaway in Killington, Vermont, call (800) 545-9407.

➤ NIA

Two of the first innovators to break from the fitness industry's cookie-cutter style of fitness were Debbie and Carlos Rosas, founders of the NIA (neuromuscular integrative action) form of movement. The Rosas were interested in helping people escape the harmful dynamics of impact aerobics. They criticized the loud, fast rock music that was deafening and impossible to shout over. They frowned upon the instructors' loud commands to "do it hard, squeeze it, hold it, tighten it." They wanted to design a class that got away from rapid, shallow breathing and fast, jerky, tense motions. They also wanted to move beyond simple-minded coordination, mindless repetition, and a total lack of body awareness.

The fact that most instructors did all of those things 12 times a week, and club members about 4 to 6 times, only reinforced the nightmare of body stress.

Skilled in a variety of movement styles such as tai chi, aikido, Feldenkrais, and aspects of authentic movement, the Rosas were aware of the dangers and shortcomings of this type of imbalanced exercise. They were shocked that people kept experiencing pain and stress from aerobics yet kept putting up with it as if it were a normal outgrowth of getting fit.

The Rosas developed a new aerobics program that integrated jazz, modern dance, yoga, and martial arts into a gentle, 60-minute class. They took their much-different NIA technique to the aerobics associations and club conventions about 10 years ago. Their nonimpact philosophy was embraced by those who were ready to abandon abusive aerobics but was questioned by the rank and file for its controversial combination of movement disciplines.

Today, the Rosas are seen as fitness experts who were ahead of their time. They now have the longest and richest background in offering holistic fitness to recovering aerobophiles. Their program is taught by licensed teachers at health clubs across the country, as well as on videotapes. For more information, contact NIA in Portland, Oregon, at (800) 762-5762.

➤ Qigong (Chi Gong)

Qi means "energy" or "life force," and *gong* means "work." When you put these two Chinese words together, you have *qigong*, a "working of energy." Although it looks a lot like tai chi, qigong offers more benefits. It's actually an ancient tool of Chinese medicine that allows you to cultivate your qi energy and experience its healing power.

In the very early stages, as you learn the simple, easy-to-follow patterns such as "dropping post" or "golden ball," you may wonder if you're missing something. You may feel that you're making small, simple movements that reap no benefits. Be patient. The real magic is in daily practice, done faithfully for years. One day, maybe a year into it, or perhaps a decade later, you'll sweep your hands through a "trembling horse" movement, and it will happen! You'll sense something more than the open space. It's a buildup of energy like a glowing snowball being pushed by your hands. Or else you'll detect a new inner sharpness and light-filled fountainhead springing out of your center. Any number of minor miracles could spring from within you.

(continued on page 140)

MY THINKING ON RUNNING

If you're already a dedicated runner, keep it up. My hat's off to you. Along with a million lifetime runners, you already know about the sport's superior advantage for maintaining a healthy weight, optimizing endurance, and building confidence. I like running because it makes me feel like a kid; there's something about the wind in my hair and the ability to propel myself faster and faster.

One of the most inspiring runs of my life was with Grete Waitz on a fun 10-K through the streets of her native Oslo, Norway. Like millions of runners, I've never been a serious competitor, but like those others, that doesn't keep me from enjoying the thrill of a big-city run. Whether you run for the endorphins or the T-shirt, you can also enjoy the time to be alone, clear your mind, energize your body, and get away from it all.

How do you start? Intersperse walking with jogging at a pace that feels good but is still a challenge. Some people find that they can alternate a minute of each, while others have to keep it down to 15 seconds. Your present fitness level, weight, and leg strength are determining factors for how long you can go.

Beginners are often alarmed that they become so short of breath so quickly. Before the cardiorespiratory benefits (such as more efficient heart pumping action and improved oxygen uptake by the working muscles) begin to kick in, beginners can fatigue rapidly with full-out runs. That's because they reach the anaerobic threshold—a state in which lactic acid, a normal by-product of metabolism, builds up in the muscles and basically shuts them down—early. If you begin with a walk-jog sequence, you can extend the duration of your exercise time, thereby building bone and muscle strength, burning calories, and increasing endurance. Walk-jog at a pace that lets you breathe evenly and converse in short sentences.

Of all sports, running is probably the easiest on your wallet. It's cheap, convenient, and fun. Your most important investment is a good pair of shoes designed for running, not for aerobics, basketball, or anything else. Some experts think that shoes are only good for 300 miles.

Depending on how many miles you clock a week, that could mean bad treads and worn-out cushioning within three months.

You should also have clothing that allows sweat to evaporate easily, and remember to drink lots of water—six to eight ounces for every 10 minutes of exercise. On hot or humid days, you may need more.

A word of caution: If you experience excessive fatigue, nausea, soreness, dizziness, or chest or arm pain while running, be sure to check with your physician before you run again. In fact, if you're over 45, haven't exercised at all, and want to take up running or any other vigorous sport, it's a good idea to have a treadmill stress test and a baseline electrocardiogram (EKG) and clearance from your doctor before you get started.

When you run, look for surfaces that provide soft landings. Streets and sidewalks are unforgiving, besides forcing you to cope with traffic and obstacles. Consistent pounding on hard surfaces can lead to overuse syndromes such as chondromalacia (aching knee joints) and shinsplints, so it's a good idea to seek out soft trails, tracks, and other kinder surfaces to give your joints and skeleton more cushioning.

How should you train? A quality training program provides you with the right amount of challenge along with adequate recovery time. If you're already enjoying a daily run, become more educated about the sport. Read *Runner's World* magazine and talk to experienced runners. Join a runner's club. Vary your runs to include speedwork, hill work, slower days, and endurance runs.

Rest, don't obsess. Runners (and cyclists) tend to be the most enthusiastic about their sports, and they often find it difficult to switch gears to other activities. Listen to your body. Take a day off at least every three days, if not every other day. You should also cross-train with weights, cycling, inline skating, or rowing. The new elliptical trainers are excellent for runners—better than steppers. Also, consider getting in the pool for some deep-water running or aqua-jogging. You will benefit from the resistance of the water without having to deal with the possible negative effects of the impact of the footstrike.

The qigong teachers I know are hesitant to describe specific moves because they know that you will experience your growing qi in your own unique way. As with all Eastern systems, a single move takes decades to master, and even then, you can continue to perfect the nuances throughout your lifetime.

Jerry Alan Johnson, Ph.D., was one of the first Westerners to intern as a doctor of advanced clinical qigong medicine at Xi Yuan Hospital in China. His videos on qigong offer a good introduction. For the best qigong exercise descriptions in print, check out Master Hong Lui's book with Paul Perry, *Mastering Miracles.* He describes how to use qigong for self-healing, longevity, and healing others.

➤ Rosen Movement

A remarkably wise teacher, Marion Rosen, now in her eighties, escaped Nazi Germany during World War II, fled to Sweden, and eventually came to the United States, where she set up shop as a physical therapist. She later developed Rosen Movement, an offshoot of her Rosen Method of Bodywork.

A classic comment from someone who has just had a Rosen bodywork session is, "I don't know what triggered it, but she just laid her hands on me very gently, and I totally let go."

I found it easy to love Rosen Movement. Instead of the instructor standing with his back to the students, as in a typical class, a Rosen teacher moves in a circle with you. Everyone has a chance to be seen, and the instructor can alter the intensity and style of the moves. The teacher, who is aware of what your body is like, can design a movement for you that makes it possible to move in a way that you never thought you could. Step by step, you become unstuck and open your mind more. This helps you become more involved in life, with more freedom and caring.

My own instructor, Mara Keller, says that Rosen has been an enormous benefit in her life, allowing her to become a good partner to herself and to others in a way "that creates not only more ease and freedom but also inner and outward harmony and creative aliveness."

Today, thousands of teachers are certified in the method. For information on classes and instructors, write to Rosen Method: The Berkeley Center, 825 Bancroft Way, Suite A, Berkeley, CA 94710, or call (800) 893-2622.

➤ Somatics

Don't be intimidated by the word or the lingo. Somatics can be difficult to understand, mainly because the discipline is packed with hard-to-decipher jargon. The word *somatic* is used in multiple ways. It can refer to a field of mind-body study and is also often used as an interchangeable professional label (such as a somatic professional or bodyworker). Simply put, though, it means "body."

Somatics as a concept encompasses many integrative mind-body models, including the work of Thomas Hanna, F. M. Alexander, Wilhelm Reich, Moshe Feldenkrais, and Ida Rolf, and methods such as Body-Mind Centering, Aston Patterning, Gestalt, Hakomi, and Sensory Awareness. The founder of the Somatics program at the California Institute of Integral Studies, Don Hanlon Johnson, is a pioneer in describing the groundwork for these various therapeutic modalities in his books *Bone, Breath, and Gesture: Practices of Embodiment*; *Groundworks: Narratives of Embodiment*; and *The Body in Psychotherapy*. Johnson is also a champion of body-oriented psychotherapy who has helped document the foundational work that has been done in various disciplines, from yoga to process-oriented psychotherapy.

An innovator in the field, Johnson describes somatics as a basic human longing to connect body processes such as your breath, movement, and sensibility with personal growth and self-awareness. Somatic practitioners help you decipher what your movement has to show you about yourself and your relationships. "They bring us closer to the wisdom inherent in the ancient structures of collagen, nerve fibers, and cerebrospinal fluid," explains Johnson.

If you are interested in learning more about somatics as a profession that you could expand into clinics, wellness programs, schools, and recovery units, write to the California Institute of Integral Studies, 1453 Mission Street, San Francisco, CA 94103.

➤ Sports Ball

Looking for a great work break that beats coffee and doughnuts? Roll around. Keep a large sports ball or medicine ball next to your desk and use it for five minutes every hour. Roll around on it to relieve lower back pain or neck problems and to release muscle tension. You can also discover ways to

STRUGGLING WITH CHANGE

While many fitness experts still thumb their noses at alternative moves, I have found plenty, like myself, who have been converted. Most of these professionals have similar stories: They grew disenchanted after failing to reach the people who "needed it most."

This disenchantment led to a professional crisis of sorts. Years of preaching only to the converted caused them to hit bottom emotionally and energetically; most of them began to question their life's work. "Am I really doing any good? Why am I doing this if no one seems to want to change?" were some of the self-reflective questions many of them posed at this critical, existential point in their careers.

To bounce back, these fitness professionals explored alternative practices. They were familiar with the popular mind-body messages of *Love, Medicine and Miracles* by Bernie Siegel, M.D.; *Minding the Body, Mending the Mind* by Joan Borysenko, Ph.D.; and *Healing Words* by Larry Dossey, M.D.; among others. In order to heal themselves, the "healers" looked to Eastern disciplines such as tai chi, yoga, aikido, acupuncture, qigong, and massage; Rosen Method Bodywork; Authentic Movement; ecstatic dance; Rolfing; Feldenkrais work; bioenergetics; the Alexander Technique; Ayurveda; macrobiotics; herbology; super-micronutrients; neopagan practices; Native American lessons; wicca; goddess spirituality; and the new multicultural slants on Buddhism, Sufism, and Taoism.

After these experiences, many reported feeling better, clearer, and more connected with their physical, emotional, and mental well-being. Deborah Kern, Ph.D., taught high-intensity aerobics for years, until she couldn't anymore. "Discovering NIA (neuromuscular integrative action) and spending my first week with the Rosas, I was completely awakened to a new relationship with my body, and I felt like I had discovered a new universe," she says. "In fact, I cried so hard after my first class; I didn't really understand the depth of my tears, how they showed me the extent of the armor I had to maintain as an instructor. Always focused on a flat ab, on a tight look. It was a toxic way to live."

Sadly, only some of these newly enlightened fitness professionals were willing to bring their broadened perspective to work. Many were reluctant to recommend their new practices to clients or others, since they felt that their fitness colleagues were too conservative and would question their involvement as bordering on quackery. Those who did step out and recommend their new mind-body adventures met with harsh resistance from the fitness industry. It is a sad state of affairs.

stretch and strengthen your hip, leg, and abdominal muscles. There are plenty of new videos and books on using these wonderful balls, which were developed in Scandinavia for athletes. Your back will love it!

Two products that you'll find in sporting goods stores are Resist-a-Ball and FlexaBall. They're often sold with videos and instruction booklets to get you started. For information on Resist-a-Ball, write to SPRI Products, Inc., 1026 Campus Drive, Mundelein, IL 60060.

➤ Stott Core Conditioning

The Stott Core Conditioning system from Toronto is one of the most effective approaches to restoring proper posture and developing a strong, stabilizing torso. Moira Stott has extensive understanding of the teachings of Joseph H. Pilates, the innovator who brought strength training to ballet artists with the hope of building strong, flexible muscles without building bulk.

The Pilates method focused on developing the deep torso strength and flexibility known as centering. Adding to the Pilates philosophy, Stott customizes her vast number of exercises to meet your needs for neuromuscular toning. She works on lengthening muscles, increasing abdominal and back strength, improving posture and body mechanics, and reducing joint and lower-back stress. You can take advantage of her system through the use of home videos and her equipment. It's like having a system based on Pilates but evolved to a higher level of effectiveness in your own home. For more information, write to 2200 Yonge Street, Suite 1402, Toronto, Ontario, Canada M4S2C6.

➤ Tai Chi

I remember being fascinated by the first news broadcasts from Beijing after President Nixon went to China. What were those graceful movements that millions of Chinese were doing in the streets of Beijing? How could something so slow be considered exercise?

Such moving meditations have been used in China for more than 2,500 years to focus the mind, strengthen the body, open energy meridians, and help the vital life force (qi) circulate. The movements, which progress from the simple to the complex, involve breathwork, balance, sustained muscular endurance, deep concentration, and coordination. Working with a tai chi master teacher, you can advance in every aspect of fitness as you practice the various moves, which often tell stories or depict natural themes.

The best way to learn tai chi is to take a class. Check your local community college, parks and recreation department, or martial arts academy.

➤ Tibetan Rites

The five Tibetan rites are yogalike exercises done by the Lamas of Tibetan monasteries, where the exercises were part of a regimen to rejuvenate the mind, body, and spirit. According to Eastern philosophy, the rites concentrate on building and aligning energy in each of the chakra points. Seven chakras, or concentrated energy centers, exist along the spine, from the tailbone to the top of the head.

The rites gained fame 60 years ago, after an elderly British colonel was brought back from death's door after learning the rites from Lamas. Later, when he returned to England, his friends failed to recognize him because he looked so youthful.

Traditional teachings suggest that each of the five positions should be repeated 21 times. I've found that this is a very strenuous practice, eliciting a great deal of heat, rapid breathing, and a fiery energy at the base of the spine. Beginners could try a more gentle approach, holding each position for a few seconds and working up to three to five repetitions at a time. Don't hold your breath with the exertion, but breathe normally throughout the exercise. Above all, it's important to perform the Five Rites in the sequence listed.

Rite 1. Standing with your arms outstretched to the sides, spin in a clockwise direction. Work up slowly to 15 complete turns. Children can do this easily because they practice like crazy. They are in touch with how much fun it is. Adults, however, don't tend to spin around and around during the normal course of the day. Consequently, the vestibular stimulators in our ears don't function as well as they once did, so we feel dizzy quickly. Don't be surprised if you can spin only a few times in the beginning. You'll eventually work up to the full 15, and your sense of balance will improve.

Rite 2. Lie on your back with your hands palms-down by your sides. Raise your head, tuck your chin into your chest, and exhale from your abdomen, tightening your belly to push out the air. Then, holding this head position, flex your feet and raise your legs from the hips until your legs are perpendicular to the floor. Your goal is to get your legs a little past a 90-degree angle. Again, this exercise is difficult for beginners with weak abdominal muscles. Work up to it slowly, maybe with one leg at a time.

Rite 3. Kneel with your legs hip-width apart and brace your hands on the backs of your thighs as you tuck your chin into your chest. Inhale and bend backward from your waist only as far as is comfortable, then let your head fall gently back. To return to the starting position, exhale and bring your head forward. The movement actually consists of one more motion, but wait until you feel comfortable with the backbend before moving on. As you progress, add this final move: Once you come back to center after bending backward, bend all the way forward from your hips, placing your forehead on the floor. As a beginner, do only one or two of these.

Rite 4. Seated on the floor with your legs outstretched in front of you, place your palms on the floor next to your hips and tuck your chin into your chest. Inhale as you bend your knees and move your hips straight up. Your knees should be at a 90-degree angle, making your body look like a table. Let your arms support most of your weight. Let your head gradually drop back. Hold. Exhale and return to the starting position.

Rite 5. Begin in a pushup position, but instead of lowering your body to the floor, raise your buttocks in the air as you push your palms into the floor. Keep your arms straight as you bring your head and chest closer to your knees. Your body should be shaped like an inverted V, with your hips at the highest point and your arms and legs outstretched and straight. Once in position, roll up onto the balls of your feet. This should look like the downward dog pose shown on page 95, except that you are on your toes. Exhale, lower your hips, and raise your chest back to the starting position.

▶ The Wave

The wave is a movement philosophy and class taught by dance innovator Gabrielle Roth, who has been a leader in ritual theater and cathartic movement for the past 30 years. Her workshops are routinely scheduled at Naropa Institute in Boulder, Colorado, Omega Institute in New York, and the Esalen Institute. This is a vigorous class that can be performed easily by anyone, no matter what their fitness level or dance experience.

Some portions of the wave are highly energizing and chaotic, while others emphasize quieter, more lyrical, flowing qualities. Roth's work is a valuable contribution to the holistic movement, restoring a sense of sacred, ecstatic dance to the average person. You can start with her workout audiocassette "Endless Wave," then graduate to "Refuge" and "Stillpoint," two of her band's recordings featuring tribal ambient music. For classes, a touring schedule, videos, and other information, write to The Moving Center, P. O. Box 2034, Red Bank, NJ 07701.

➤ World-Beat Workout

International teacher Kristi Rudolph designed this embodied dance program for fitness studios as a personal gesture of her own healing. Way back when, Rudolph got swept up in the fitness craze, teaching a huge, unhealthy number of classes a week to the very fit in structured settings. After years of abusing her own body, Rudolph ached for a return to embodied dance and spent one summer traveling across Africa, dancing to drums and sleeping on the earth. When she returned, she couldn't teach the same way anymore.

Interested in creating a safe environment for self-exploration and change for herself and her clients, she brought respect, growth, and sacredness into the fitness studio. "World-beat workout is not about dance but about dancing," Rudolph explains. "We are not thinking from a Western perspective of achievement and performance but from a spiritual sense of enjoyment and community." Working with five principles—controlled relaxation, a lower center of gravity, moving from the heart, moving together as a group, and rhythm—Rudolph teaches other instructors how to duplicate her programs at No Sweat Studios in Albany, California. Classes with world-beat music, tribal drumming, and jazz fusion rhythms are being offered in major clubs nationwide. Based on my travels and phone calls, I've found that the name of the class changes at each club, but the underlying method is usually the same.

➤ Yoga

I have profound respect for yoga as a 5,000-year-old path to spiritual enlightenment, and as such, I have a hard time seeing it depicted as a "killer aerobic" workout or a "mega-stretching" routine. Nevertheless, that is exactly its appeal for millions today. Walk into any urban fitness center, and you'll find that yoga has become one of the most popular classes in our stress-ridden society. As one fitness director told me, "I can't fill my step classes, but yoga is packed."

Be that as it may, I've grown to realize that the ancient and traditional yoga will survive this latest trendy spin, and some of the more esoteric benefits will still seep into unsuspecting practitioners bit by bit. The truth is that most people don't really consider yoga to be anything more than a series of postures for relaxation or a power-building workout, and true followers of an authentic yogic path are rarely seen or heard from.

True to our go-for-the-gusto way of life in the West, we've developed our own abridged form of Ashtanga yoga called Power Yoga. Who teaches Power Yoga? As a journalist, I was asked to cover one yoga "star" whose experience with the Eastern discipline was minimal but whose status as a former Wilhelmina model was meant to quicken my pulse.

This type of popularization makes long-standing yoga teachers like Rodney Yee, Lilias, and Richard Freeman cringe. Nevertheless, they are happy to see yoga—in any form—making strong headway.

Rather than going to a big-city gym that will be more likely to teach the more aggressive and less mindful Power Yoga, look for classes at yoga centers. There you will find different forms of yoga, such as:

- Iyengar, which puts the emphasis on careful execution and form.
- Kripalu, which can be quite strenuous because postures are held for a long time.
- Hatha, which is the simplest and most accessible type for beginners.
- Ashtanga, which is a fast-paced, heated form of yoga that in India is taught to the young and those with a lot of energy.

It is easy to find out more about this deeply spiritual discipline. There are plenty of good books and videos available, and dedicated yoga institutes are common in big cities. Even some health-club classes can be worthwhile ways for getting you started and directed.

9

Gather 30 as You Go

Throughout this book, I've railed against tired, repetitive aerobics classes, hard-core workouts, and expensive exercise equipment. I've done so at the risk of alienating a few of you, the few who make up the 2 out of 10 people who find the routine of going to a gym, taking the same aerobics class, or working out several times a week on a treadmill or stationary cycle completely acceptable. In fact, you enjoy it.

That doesn't mean that you've tapped into your fitness instinct, though, and it doesn't mean that your fitness routine doesn't need some adjusting. Even if you're a true diehard who practices unwavering discipline no matter what the obstacles, you can benefit from a change of pace. Even if you don't think you need variety, your body does. Here are a number of reasons why.

- Rote, repetitious movement can become boring. No matter how strong your discipline is now, you'll eventually have trouble sticking with it.
- Doing the same type of movement every day can lead to overuse injuries. Your body was made to move in many different directions. When you force it to do the same thing over and over, you wear down cartilage and tear your muscles and tendons.
- Lack of variety reduces your calorie burn. Once your body has mastered a movement, it doesn't need to work as hard to keep doing it.
- Repetitive motion underchallenges your brain. Basically, you don't have to think or try as hard to do the routine. This can foster rigidity of thinking and

brain function, eventually leading to a lower IQ and less creativity. The more neural connections your brain makes, and the more brain cells that fire, the more opportunity there is for creative new solutions, flexible thinking, and psychological adaptability—all important aspects of countering premature aging. A study of senior exercisers showed that the group that was asked to come up with their own creative choreography inundated more areas of their brain with oxygen and activity than the group that simply followed the leader.

CHOOSE WHAT WORKS FOR YOU

While most people agree that nothing beats the fit life for overall health and stamina, not everyone is willing to commit to the same conditioning routine. "Being fit" means different things to different folks, and there is an optimal level of fitness for every body.

For some, striving for fitness means saying good-bye to their sedentary lifestyles and reducing their risks of disease while achieving lasting mental and physical health benefits. For others, fitness means high athletic functioning, complete with rippling physiques and super-charged sports performance. Whatever your starting point, you have a multitude of options and techniques before you, all making the fit life accessible and enjoyable.

Two different styles have emerged on the fitness landscape over the past few years. One you may already be familiar with is aimed at high-level fitness; the other is a new recommendation called moderate activity that is designed to entice more people to the fit life.

For details of the first approach, see "High-Level Fitness." It's meant for the 20 percent of us who are already dedicated to frequent exercise. For those of us who don't aspire to athletic greatness or rippling muscles, there is the moderate approach. That is the program outlined in chapter 7, in which you do a few moments of movement each and every hour based on your fitness personality.

No matter what style you choose, the most comprehensive program for overall fitness tackles each of the primary components: aerobics for cardio-respiratory function, weight training for muscular strength and endurance, and stretching for improved flexibility.

THE POWER OF MODERATE ACTIVITY

Convinced for so long of the value of the conventional exercise prescription, few experts could believe that smaller, shorter periods of exercise accomplished throughout the day would do any good. To put the idea to the test, experts at the Cooper Institute for Aerobics Research in Dallas put 235 people into two exercise groups: one doing lifestyle activities, and the other doing structured workouts. The workout group used the institute's gym and indoor track, stair steppers, and treadmills. The lifestyle group did no workouts on

HIGH-LEVEL FITNESS

This is the "gold standard" approach to fitness training, and it requires top-priority dedication. That's right—a no-excuses mindset. (If you haven't already guessed, this isn't my favorite method. I'm mentioning it, however, because it does work for some people who are intuitively motivated by athletic pursuits.)

If you love to play sports, you should consider the following routine to avoid injuries or the overuse syndrome that you often encounter when you merely strut your stuff as a weekend warrior.

Aerobics
Type: Walking, running, cycling, swimming, or dancing.
Intensity: 60 to 90 percent of your maximum heart rate.
Duration: 20 to 60 minutes.
Frequency: Three to five times a week.

Strength Training
Type: Weights, resistance machines, or calisthenics.
Intensity: Enough repetitions to fatigue the muscle.
Duration: 20 to 30 minutes, working each major muscle group.
Frequency: Two or three times a week.

Flexibility Training
Type: Yoga, stretching, or other flexibility routines.
Intensity: Hold each stretch at a point of mild tension for 10 to 20 seconds.
Duration: 10 to 15 minutes, working each major muscle group.
Frequency: Five to seven times a week.

Numerous books written during the past two decades provide abundant rationales, research, and data that support this type of regimen. Once again, it's excellent for the 20 percent of you who manage to follow it consistently.

equipment but were counseled to walk, golf, dance, stride, cycle, play with kids, climb stairs, garden, or do a number of other enjoyable things. The only requirement was that the activity should force them to pick up their breathing and work their muscles a little.

To everyone's surprise, at the end of the study, the two groups had similar muscle gains and fat losses. Also, although the workout group had a higher treadmill score, the lifestyle group burned about the same number of calories throughout the day.

Hard-core fitness fanatics often think that this gentler approach is too lightweight. It's not. In these well-documented studies, the new moderate activity guidelines for fitness proved to be just as beneficial for overall health and longevity as the "gold standard" approach. Also, since the traditional exercise recommendation tends to be more complicated and time-consuming, fewer people actually follow it. Here's how to make short bursts work for you.

A DAY IN THE LIFE OF HOWARD

I want to tell you the story of Howard, a guy who was completely invested in the "gold standard" of exercise throughout his years in college. He faithfully exercised three times a week for an hour at a time.

Then he got a job. His career started to skyrocket, and suddenly the "gold standard" began to tarnish. Here's his typical day.

Early in the morning, he bargains with his snooze alarm for the last minute of sleep, then gives up and stumbles out of bed. There's no time for breakfast, so he eats on the run, grabbing a couple of mega-muffins on the way to work. Once there, he rides an elevator to the 19th floor and enters his cubicle. He sits in his chair, turns on the computer, reads his e-mail, listens to his voice-mail, opens his snail mail, and gets to work.

He picks up lunch from a fast-food place and stuffs down a super-size "value" meal, a total of maybe 1,200 calories.

He returns to work, where he spends the rest of the day sitting, except for taking a couple of elevator rides and a few jaunts to the copy machine. At the end of the day, he packs some paperwork in his briefcase, walks the short distance to the parking lot, and begins his 45-minute drive home.

Gather 30 as you go. Accumulate 30 minutes or more of moderate physical activity throughout the course of your day. The hourly movement program outlined in chapter 7 is a great way to do this, and it's what I recommend most. But it's not the only way. You can do three 10-minute sessions a day, or one 30-minute movement sequence, or maybe even 15 sessions of 2 minutes each. Just about any combination that results in 30 cumulative minutes will work to lower your total cholesterol, boost your healthy high-density lipoprotein (HDL) cholesterol, and slash levels of artery-clogging low-density lipoprotein (LDL) cholesterol. In any case, my recommendation is that you incorporate small workouts into every day. Quicken your pulse, feel a flush of heat and energy, and even get a bit dewy.

Keep the intensity moderate. Aim to burn at least 4.5 calories a minute as you do these short bursts. That's about the intensity of a brisk walk, gardening, walking the dog, or cycling on level terrain. Some other ideas: hiking, dancing,

---

He thinks that he'll try to ride his bike for a while at home, then remembers that he has to finish up a conference call in an hour. He stops at a Chinese takeout restaurant and orders some dinner to go—fried sweet-and-sour pork and four egg rolls. He drives home, parks in the garage, walks into his apartment, and grabs a soda. He opens his briefcase on the table and positions the phone and his papers so he's ready for his call. Seated, he conducts his business on the phone, leafs through his papers, and eats dinner at the same time.

After the call, he realizes that his favorite show is on TV. He thinks about dragging his bike out of the apartment, but when he considers the traffic on the city streets and the darkening hour, he passes on it.

Problem: Howard can't squeeze in his old exercise routine any more, so he winds up doing nothing, eating more, and gaining weight. Any one of us could easily relate to Howard's story. Because we don't admit the truth of our hectic schedules, we stay nailed into the coffin of a routine that is impossible to pull off.

Solution: If, every hour of every day, Howard could move with stretches, strengthening, and "gather 30 as you go" aerobics, he could increase his total daily calorie expenditure to 2,100 calories. If he improved his eating habits as well, he could stop the insidious weight gain and maintain a healthy level of strength, flexibility, and endurance.

running up and down stairs, washing the car, physical play with youngsters (especially toddlers), vigorous housework, yardwork, or recreational games—anything that involves moving your body in large, rhythmic patterns that are out of your ordinary scope.

Have a good time. Make sure that you're doing some type of exercise (try calling it movement or play instead) that you thoroughly enjoy, and that you approach it in a relaxed frame of mind. A do-or-die attitude about exercise may block its positive benefits.

STRENGTHENING PROGRAMS

A lot of mainstream fitness experts will tell you about the benefits of lifting weights. I agree with them 100 percent: Getting stronger is a good thing. I don't necessarily agree with their methods, however.

First, the benefits. When your body grows stronger, it delights you in unexpected ways. Compare periods in your life when you've been physically strong with those when you've been weaker. There is a poise, confidence, and grace that accompanies strength. It's a quiet reserve, a peace of mind that comes from knowing that you can count on your body.

Within a few weeks of starting a strength-training program, you can clearly appreciate the gains in muscle strength and endurance, because common tasks such as opening a jar, lifting two bags of groceries, or moving a computer monitor get a little easier. Here are some other benefits.

More fat burning. If you're really consistent with a weight-training routine, either at the gym or with some calisthenics at home, you move beyond those small gains to one of the most important benefits of strength training: Your fat-burning capacity increases.

Within about three months, your body's muscle-to-fat ratio will improve, and you will start to burn calories more efficiently. Every time you perform a strengthening routine, you challenge the lean muscle in your body to increase in size and functional capacity. Your muscles actually get "smarter" in their ability to use fat and burn it up.

Less risk of premature aging. Loss of strength is the single most tragic reason for age-related functional loss, curtailed activities, diminished capacity, and even a shrinking skeleton. If you don't consciously use a muscle, you begin to lose it, and this loss occurs at an accelerated rate once you're over 40.

We all lose muscle as we age—unless we decide not to. It's really that simple. Muscle mass peaks at around age 30. If we pay no attention to retaining it, we lose about five to six pounds of muscle every decade after that. At this rate, when we reach our midseventies, we're left with about two-thirds of the muscle that we had when we were 20. Because muscle is metabolically active tissue, there is a corresponding decrease in our resting metabolism, and we burn fewer calories at rest. That's why 40-year-olds complain about gaining weight more easily than they did at 30, and why 50-year-olds complain even louder.

CHANGE YOUR MINDSET

People sometimes motivate themselves by wondering, "Have I been exercising long enough to burn off that dessert?" *Warning*: Don't go there. This kind of calculation is ultimately depressing. No doubt you've seen calorie-burning charts: They're made up of rows of numbers that represent the calories expended for a long list of exercises and then compare those numbers with the calories ingested from foods like pizza, fries, and frozen yogurt. When you really consider how long and hard you have to work out in order to erase the fattening effects of a single slice of mud pie, it's enough to make you say "The heck with it," and order a double.

Let me give you some examples. In order to burn the calories from one fried chicken sandwich from McDonald's, you'd have to walk on a treadmill at 3.5 miles per hour for 20 hours. To burn the equivalent of one mocha cappuccino with whipped cream, you would have to stay on the Stairmaster for 22 hours.

If you think of cardiovascular exercise as simply a calorie-crunching, fat-burning endeavor, it will soon grow to be as dull and lifeless as taking out the garbage. That's the bad news. Here's the good news. Your normal waking metabolism, which includes all of the caloric energy necessary for breathing, moving about, digestion, light activity, and even resting and sleeping, is your biggest calorie burner, not exercise. If you weigh 130 pounds, you burn about 1,650 calories a day just for normal activities.

Knowing that, why not switch gears and make your workouts fun? Find an aerobics class with some interesting new twists. Let a power walk at lunch double as a means of blowing off steam with a co-worker. Take your first inline skating lesson. Join a doubles tennis league. Do it because you love it.

Lower risk of osteoporosis. Strength training prevents this number one disability for millions of older women by keeping calcium in the bones. By using weight-bearing exercise, a calcium supplement of 1,000 to 1,200 milligrams a day, and natural hormones from sources such as soybeans and yams, many women have been able to retain bone strength.

A better appearance. Miriam Nelson, Ph.D., is a scientist at the Jean Mayer USDA Human Nutrition Research Center on Aging at Tufts University in Boston. She studied a group of women ages 50 to 70 for one year as they participated in a twice-weekly weight-training program using light dumbbells. At the end of the year, the women were 75 percent stronger, their balance had improved by 14 percent, and they had increased bone density. The women also lost three pounds of fat and gained the same amount of muscle, but since muscle takes up less space than fat, they were able to wear smaller-size clothing.

Easier movement. These numbers all sound good, but the real proof that strength training is worthwhile is what it did for the women in studies: They became more active in general, enjoying gardening, skating, dancing, horseback riding, and other fun activities that they had never done before.

One problem with strength training as it's traditionally taught to people is that it takes a lot of time. Fitness experts often tell you to use dumbbells, either at a gym or at home, and complete 10 to 15 different exercises, often doing each one two or three times. Not only is this time-consuming, it's boring.

Fortunately, there's another, better approach: Try strength training the intuitive way.

Throughout the day, your body sends you messages to strengthen, move, flex, and stretch your muscles. If you're used to ignoring those signals, it's going to take some effort for you to become alert to them, but you can do it.

The idea is to make it fun and instinctual. Simply apply the "gather 30 as you go" concept to strength training. I've already provided you with several strengthening exercises in chapter 7. To offer you more variety, here are four additional strengthening sequences that you can integrate into your day. Try them for a while, based on your abilities and available time. As you do the exercises, however, you may find that your body is urging you to move in different ways. Go with those urges. They're your fitness instinct talking to you loud and clear.

EASIEST (5 to 10 Minutes)

- 12 pushups (See page 99.)
- 12 gluteal squeezes
  (Just squeeze your buttocks together.)
- 10 lunges (See page 100.)
- 6 to 8 chair dips
  (See page 118.)
- 12 shoulder shrugs (Hold a light dumbbell or heavy bottle in each hand and shrug your shoulders up toward your ears, then back down.)
- 12 lateral arm raises (Hold light dumbbells at your sides, then slowly lift them until your arms are parallel to the floor, with your hands at shoulder height. Lower and repeat.)

INTERMEDIATE (15 to 30 Minutes)

Do two sets of 10 to 14 repetitions of each exercise. In time, work up to three sets. Do workout 1, then do workout 2 a day or two later.

WORKOUT 1: UPPER BODY
- Bicep curls (With your arms down at your sides, hold a light dumbbell or heavy bottle in each hand, palms forward. One at a time, bend your elbows and bring the weight up to shoulder level, then lower it.)
- Tricep curls (Raise your arms over your head, palms facing forward. Slowly bend your arms at the elbows so that your forearms and hands fall behind your head, then slowly raise them. When you feel comfortable with the motion, do it while holding a light dumbbell or heavy bottle with both hands.)
- Wrist curls (Holding a light dumbbell or heavy can in each hand, move your hands up and down from the wrists.)
- Front and lateral arm raises (Lateral raises are described above. A front arm raise is essentially the same, except that you lift the dumbbell in front of you rather than at your side.)
- Inclined bench row (This is good for your back. Put your right knee on a sturdy chair, grip the back of the chair with

(continued)

your right hand, and lean forward slightly. Hold a light dumbbell or can in your left hand and let it dangle straight down toward the floor. Next, bring the weight up to your chest and then lower. Switch sides and repeat.)

• Bench press (This works your chest, shoulders, and triceps. Lying on your back on a bench, hold a light dumbbell in each hand near your armpits. Press the weights upward until your arms are extended overhead. Return to the starting position.)

• Abdominal curls or crunches (See page 109.)

WORKOUT 2: LOWER BODY

• Leg press or squats (See page 105.)

• Step-ups (Do these as described on page 118, but hold a light dumbbell or heavy can in each hand, and lead with the same leg for a full set.)

• Lunges (See page 100.)

• Leg extensions (Sit on a ledge or on a chair from which your feet do not touch the floor. With your back straight, raise your lower legs until they are parallel to the floor. Slowly return them to the starting position, then repeat. Your upper body should stay still during the exercise. In time, you can try some ankle weights for greater strengthening.)

• Hamstring curls (Lie on your stomach on a table, bed, or counter so that your knees and lower legs are just off the edge. Bend your knees and raise your heels until your lower legs are perpendicular to the surface you're lying on. Lower your legs slowly and repeat. Again, doing this with ankle weights will make you stronger.)

• Hip extensions (See page 162.)

• Calf raises (Stand with your legs together and your feet flat on the floor, then rise up on your toes.)

• Abdominal curls or crunches (See page 109.)

> ### TOUGHEST (30 Minutes or More)
>
> This program mixes upper and lower body exercises into one long, hard routine. For each exercise, do two sets of 10 to 14 repetitions. In time, work up to three sets.
>
> - Squats (See page 105.)
> - Lunges (See page 100.)
> - Abdominal curls or crunches (See page 109.)
> - Bicep curls (See page 157.)
> - Wrist curls (See page 157.)
> - Tricep curls (See page 157.)
> - Lateral arm raises (See page 157.)
> - Bench presses (See page 158.)
> - Leg extensions (See page 158.)
> - Hamstring curls (See page 158.)
> - Shoulder shrugs (See page 157.)
> - Back extensions (Lying face-down on the floor, lift your head and upper chest. Hold for four to six seconds before lowering, using only the muscles of your lower back.)
> - Calf raises (See page 158.)

DISCOVER THE JOYS OF STRETCHING

Most people go after a stretch as if they're trying to win a tug-of-war, as if force were going to accomplish something. I want you to rethink stretching so thoroughly that you start to move like a cat. That way, you'll tap into your flexibility instinct. Once again, if you're used to sitting still for long hours, never adjusting your posture and ignoring the moment-by-moment proddings of your body to stretch, it's going to take a little while for you to become aware of this. You can, though, so hang in there.

The more you stretch throughout the day, the more you'll become aware of your body's natural proddings to maintain flexibility by putting your muscles and joints through their full ranges of motion. Moreover, you'll accrue the benefits of frequent stretching: less muscle tension, less stiffness, better elasticity of the muscles and tendons, and a reduced risk of injuries.

Conventional exercise routines recommend that you stretch after an aerobics or strengthening routine. It's far better for you to take a one-minute stretch break every hour rather than just two or three times a week. As you stretch, keep the following tips in mind.

BECOME A LEAN FAN OF FIDGETING

Fidgeting is the key to why some people don't gain weight even when they overeat, according to research done at the Mayo Clinic in Rochester, Minnesota. Researchers studied 16 people who overate. They found that the key factor in predicting fat gain was the difference in calories burned during the normal activities of daily living. People who fidgeted, moved around, changed position often, and so on were able to keep their weights stable.

The 16 volunteers gained an average of 10 pounds in the two months of the study, but actual weight gain varied from 2 pounds to almost 16 pounds. Those with the greatest increase in fidgeting gained the least fat. In some cases, the fidgeters burned off as many as 692 calories per day through what scientists call NEAT, or nonexercise activity thermogenesis.

The moral: The latest weight-loss secret is to move around like a little child with ants in his pants. Move, move, move. Change your position. Stretch and strengthen. Learn to fidget or learn to dance. It's all romance to your body.

Be gentle. Intensity is counterproductive to stretching. A sudden, fast, or forceful stretch will elicit a reflex that triggers an instantaneous contraction. Muscles are lengthened by gentle coaxing. As you stretch, you should think, "I get a lot more accomplished with gentleness."

Be fluid. Enter and exit your stretch with fluidity. Keep your mind on the stretch, inviting your muscles to lengthen and release toxins, to loosen and widen the space between the fibers, thus inviting in oxygen and nutrients. Think, "I am feeding my muscles with everything they need."

Be patient. It takes 10 seconds for a muscle to give up trying to contract when a stretch is applied. It takes another 10 seconds for it to be convinced to let go and ease up. The following 10 seconds are spent in lengthening. After doing each of the stretches that begin on the opposite page, return to the pre-stretch position for a few seconds of rest to help blood flow into the area. Stretching correctly is a waiting game, so make sure that your mind and your breathing are well-occupied. Wonderful things happen to those who can stretch for a full minute. Think, "This muscle gives me 24 hours of on-call duty. I can give it a minute of bliss."

Make the most of your stretch. What else can you do during a long stretch?

- Massage your face muscles with frequent yawns, opening your jaw and releasing the tension there.
- Hum your favorite ditty, chant, or love song into your stretching muscles. Vibrations are good medicine. They set up a calming action and remind you to take deep breaths.
- As you're stretching, tighten your abdomen with quick contractions and say "Ha!" like a sudden laugh. You may trigger a full belly laugh, which will assist further letting go in the muscles. Laughter is the elixir of release.
- Visualize your breath entering the stretched area, helping it unwind.

Be consistent. Don't stretch just a few times a week. Don't stretch just once a day. Stretching is something that should happen every hour on the hour. It already does as you sleep—you're just not aware of it. To get an idea of how often you should stretch, watch a cat for a few hours. Cats stretch before they eat (a prehunt warmup), after they eat, before they lie down, after they wake up, and anytime they start to move. Whether it's a simple post-sports routine or a yoga class, stretching adds suppleness and fluidity and maintains a full range of motion, while it also clears your mind and centers your focus. It also helps minimize injuries and coax out the kinks from a previous workout.

Get warm. Never stretch cold muscles. Always warm up for five minutes first with some rhythmic movement.

Here are some one-minute stretches to do throughout the day; do them on a mat or carpeted floor.

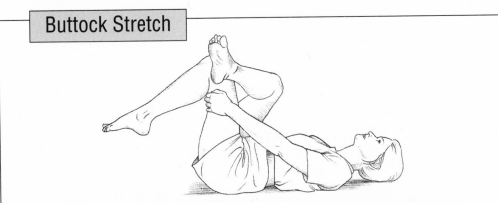

Buttock Stretch

Lie on your back with your left leg bent and place your right ankle on your left knee. Place your hands behind your left thigh for support and gently pull your knee toward your chest. Hold for 30 seconds, then switch leg positions and repeat.

Hip Stretch

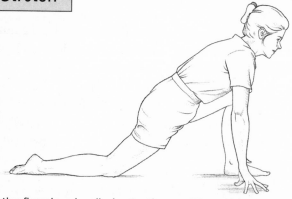

Kneel on the floor in a hurdler's starting position, with your left leg bent at a right angle under your chest and your hands on the floor supporting your torso. Extend your right leg behind you and place your knee on the floor. (You can place a towel or mat under your knee for comfort.) You should feel the stretch in the front of your right thigh, all the way up toward the top of the hip joint in your groin. Hold for 30 seconds, then repeat with your right leg bent and your left extended.

Achilles Tendon and Calf Stretch

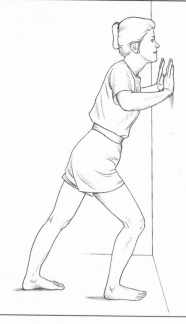

Stand facing a wall and place your hands against it. Place one foot behind the other with the toes pointing forward and lean toward the wall. Alternatively, you can press your toes against the bottom of a tree or wall. Hold for 30 seconds, then switch leg positions and repeat.

Quadriceps Stretch

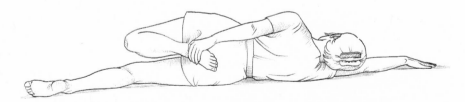

Lie on your right side with your legs together and your head resting on your out-stretched arm. Bend your left leg, then grasp your foot and pull it gently up toward your back. Hold for 30 seconds, then lie on your left side and repeat.

Hamstring Stretch

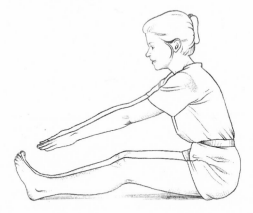

Sit on the floor with your legs extended in front of you and your knees slightly bent. Extend your arms and gently reach for your toes, bending your torso toward your knees. Hold for 30 seconds.

Lower Back Stretch

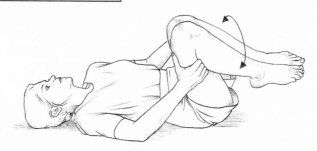

Lie on your back with your knees bent, then bring them toward your chest. For a higher back stretch, let your knees fall to one side and then the other. Hold each position for 30 seconds.

Chest Stretch

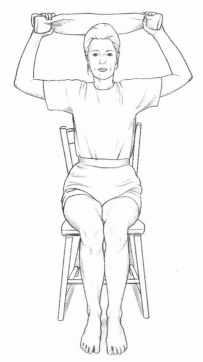

Sit in a chair with both feet flat on the floor. Hold one end of a towel in each hand and stretch it in front of you. Keeping the towel stretched taut, raise it over your head, then bend your elbows and slowly lower it behind you as far as you can. Hold the stretch for 30 seconds.

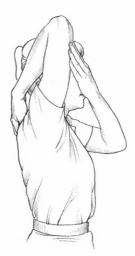

Triceps Stretch

Raise your right arm over your head, then bend your elbow, reach down your back, and finger-walk your hand down your spine. Assist the stretch with your other hand by pushing your elbow back. Hold for 30 seconds, then switch arm positions and repeat.

MAKE AEROBICS FUN AGAIN

Maybe it's time to leave those leotards behind and try a totally different approach to aerobics. After all, you don't need to burn all those calories and "feel the burn" in one long session. Instead, you can do short bursts of multiple aerobic activities throughout the day. The method works for a number of reasons,

It taps into your fitness instinct. Your body was not designed to "work out" for a rare hour here and there and be sedentary in between. Rather, it was designed to move continuously throughout the day. Every time you try to force yourself to keep moving for minutes upon minutes, your body rebels—and so does your mind.

It's convenient. Because you're moving for such a short amount of time, you don't work up a sweat. Thus, you rarely need to change clothes or even take a shower. You can work these short, 5- to 10-minute movement sessions into breaks at work or at home.

You'll look forward to it. Mini-exercise breaks boost your mood and increase your energy levels. Pretty soon you'll find that you won't be able to get along without them. Try short sessions of any of the following activities.

- A brisk walk
- Jumping jacks
- A 10-minute run
- Dancing to your favorite song
- Riding a bike around the block a couple of times
- Yardwork or housework
- Playing with children
- Chasing your dog around the yard
- Walking up a few flights of stairs
- Marching in place

The old jump-up-and-down aerobics class of the early 1980s is worn at the edges, and for good reason. It's hard on the joints and boring for the mind. Some hot new trends, however, are showing up in aerobics classes nationwide, and they're gathering converts. If you are driven to exercise for 30 minutes or more at a time, I recommend these classes because they do tap into some of our natural instincts.

People who love aerobics classes enjoy group exercise to music, the social network, the energy generated by new teachers and fresh material, and just being in synch as they march out a cadence with other aerobicizers. Because these classes have been around for at least 20 years, many loyal fans, both men and women, are experiencing a never-before-known confidence in their bodies. They are willing to take a step toward unfamiliar territory and are stretching their bodies and their imaginations to new rhythms from around the world.

Aerobics classes that stay within safe and sane guidelines move your body in nonjarring ways along proper biomechanical lines. This new breed of classes departs from the traditional by moving improvisationally, using your body to its fullest range of motion and grooving energetically with all its parts—rib cage, hips, torso, head, and shoulders—not just your arms and legs. For instance, Paula Moreschi founded Physical Culture, an alternative fitness center in Seattle that plays not Top 40 tunes but "underground" rock music. With help from ethnic and street dance, martial arts, body sculpting, yoga, drama, and classical dance, the classes teach students to let go of inhibitions and free their bodies. Here are 15 other new, more intuitive types of aerobics classes.

➤ Asian Power Class

Research the basic moves of a beginning martial arts or self-defense classes, throw in a good measure of tai chi for grace and agility, and bill the class as the latest import from the Pacific Rim. Make it a class that not only helps you get in shape but could also help save your life, and you have the main components of Asian Power workouts.

➤ The Big Easy

Similar to traditional aerobics, these classes are popping up all over and are catering to people who want moderation. The moves are interesting, although slower-paced. The target heart rates for these classes are as low as 50 to 55 percent, which is my general recommendation for holistic fitness. It's a class that underwhelms, and because it gets the discouraged beginner past the number one hurdle—early fatigue—it works especially well for those who previously have been reluctant to take aerobics. This method takes the strain out of exercise and puts the pleasure back in.

➤ Body Sculpting

This is not just a low-impact-with-weights class, it's toning with the intention to reshape your body: a more intense, slower-paced, higher-resistance class with a target heart rate usually under 50 percent. One version, called Body Pump, involves rhythmic weight training set to music and uses a step and lighter weights.

To be ready for this intensity, you should be able to perform 16 repetitions without fatigue. Be sure that you don't let the music push you into performing the moves at too fast a clip, otherwise you'll risk injury to tendons, joints, and ligaments. Long warmups are essential for this class.

➤ Boxing

Now undergoing a surge of interest, boxing classes are billed as cardiobox, martial arts boxing, kickboxing, and other variants. Since they offer very high intensity with simple, repetitive moves, classes are often very gender balanced. Some instructors rely on lots of equipment such as bags and gloves, while others can put you through the paces with no equipment.

➤ Gotta Dance

Due to a demand from long-time aerobics participants for something a lot more fun and useful, there is an interesting transition from aerobics to almost-dance that's occurring in many clubs. Learning hot new moves in the aerobics studio lets you show off your stuff on the weekend dance floor. If you're ready to abandon straight aerobics for something more swinging, look for an instructor who will help you build slowly to more complicated dance steps by starting with a simple pattern. This will keep frustration to a minimum and allow you to learn as the class progresses.

➤ Group Strength Training

Some instructors are choreographing strength-training classes to music and using various kinds of equipment, such as steps, Power Boards, bands, and weights, to challenge specific muscle groups.

➤ Indoor Cycling Classes and Spinning

Too tough for beginners, Spinning classes were conceived by fitness trainer Johnny G as a guided indoor stationary bike tour. Since then, a new generation of indoor cycling classes has been spawned. They are excellent for aerobics enthusiasts who want to be pushed to new heights. It's still important, though, to find an instructor who lets you stay in charge of your training intensity.

As you're Spinning, you visualize yourself on cross-country terrain, sometimes standing on the pedals to push uphill and then getting some high-speed cruising breaks without resistance. Unfortunately, these classes are available only at clubs that have the space and can afford the bikes.

➤ The Method

Dancer and fitness trainer Cal Pozo created the Method, a system of physical conditioning that promotes mental and physical harmony through a series of interconnected movements. It includes tai chi, yoga, dance, and the deep muscle work of Pilates and Feldenkrais. Pozo sees most fitness workouts as too fragmented and believes that dancers have been integrating different kinds of techniques into their training to keep their muscles challenged, to diversify the movement, and to prevent boredom. The Method is taught in more than 500 studios and is available on a series of videos from the Physicalmind Institute in Santa Fe, New Mexico.

THE FITNESS PYRAMID

Here's yet another reason that it's so hard to stick to a fitness routine: Many of us are so out of touch with what our bodies really need and with our natural urges to move that we force ourselves to move in unnatural ways. When our bodies are craving stretching, we inflict aerobics upon them. When they're craving some brisk movement, we do leg lifts instead.

Here's a quick and easy way to get back in touch with your natural urges and needs. Think of the different types of movement you do during your waking hours—daily lifestyle activities, aerobics, strength training, stretching, and rest. Next, assign times to them and stack them up as a pyramid.

Here's how it should stack up, according to the American College of Sports Medicine (ACSM), which created the Physical Activity Pyramid to help people understand how much exercise they really need.

The base of the pyramid, and thus the largest level, represents lifestyle activities, such as walking (not driving), using the stairs (not the elevator), and doing housework and yardwork. Your body craves at least 30 minutes of active movement almost every day of the week.

The next, somewhat smaller level is active aerobics or sports. Because activities such as step aerobics and tennis involve a boost in heart rate, they can be performed less often. You should strive for 20 minutes of aerobic movement three to six days a week.

The third and next-smallest level includes stretching and strengthening. Stretching is great for your body, but it takes very little time. In a few minutes, you can effectively stretch most of your major muscle groups. The ACSM recommends stretching as often as every day, and so do I. As for strengthening, it takes only a short time to put muscles through a good workout, then they need two days to recuperate, so exercise each major muscle group only two or three times a week.

At the peak of the pyramid, representing the smallest chunk of time, is inactivity. Given the time spent sleeping, eating, and doing other necessarily inactive things such as working or paying bills, your physical body needs a minimum of extra idle time. Thus, time spent watching TV or reading the newspaper, while potentially relaxing for your mind, offers little of value to your physical body.

➤ Power Board

Jeff Tuller, president of Power Board, is hoping that his springy step plat-form will take off and become as big as Spinning. The rebound quality of the board is a great shock absorber for anybody who wants to give their knees a rest, and it's kind of fun. You can attach cords to the board and use it for resis-tance training or simply bounce away for a cardio workout.

➤ Restorative Fitness

This is the brainchild of exercise innovator Nancy Minges, a director at the Claremont Resort and Spa in Oakland, California. With a master's degree in holistic health, certification in Continuum, and experience in authentic move-ment, Minges has redefined aerobic programming in her club to a twenty-first-century, higher standard. Her class schedule reads like a menu of delectable fitness treats: mindful stretching, undercurrents, restorative stretch, core power, world-beat, active yoga, and so on. She and her staff of trainers—including David Parker, who combines practical tips from the world of physical therapy with the best of athletic training—are available for consultation. Contact the Claremont Resort at (800) 551-7266.

➤ Rock Video Classes

Hams, fans, and star performers come out in the open and on camera during this big-screen class. Instructors teach participants all types of funky, hip-hop dance moves that offer lots of toning potential for the abs, buttocks, thighs, and calves. Usually, two or three home video cameras are set up on tripods in the protected corners of a class, and the footage is shown simultane-ously on large monitors. Class participants get a kick out of watching each other. David Gray innovated this new angle, and sports expos have also played with this rock aerobics concept.

➤ Sufi Dancing

Called Sufi dancing in some cities and just free dance in others, this is a form of wild and creative dance with driving rhythms (sometimes sacred chants) and good, heartfelt vibes. People dance by themselves, then join in large circles to close the session.

The sessions are always smoke-free and alcohol-free, and they're often done barefoot. Participants pay a nominal fee (about $5) to dance in a safe, nonjudg-mental atmosphere. I know of several places that offer this type of dancing, including Dance Place in Santa Monica, California; Dance Jam in Austin, Texas; and Dance Spirit in New York City. If there's not one in your town, start one.

➤ Trekking

What do you do with a room full of treadmills? Start a class that exercises to music. Trekking is the brainchild of Jefferson Hills of StarTrac by Unisen. Led by an instructor who coaches them to change elevation and speed for a challenging treadmill workout, participants are still able to personalize their routines for their own abilities. Trekking premiered at the 1998 convention of the International Health, Racquet, and Sportsclub Association, a national organization of fitness clubs, and will make its appearance at more health clubs during the next few years.

➤ World-Beat Classes

I mentioned these classes in chapter 8, but they're so much fun that I encourage diehard aerobics fans to try them, too. There's an entire world of movement and expression to choose from. The hottest classes are in cities with large, diverse ethnic mixes, such as Miami, New York, and Los Angeles. Have you considered Afro-Caribbean moves and rhythms? There's also an exciting class in Atlanta that features an instructor teaching jazz-African gospel. The moves play off the downbeat and swing low in an Earth-connected style. Some classes offer live musicians and drummers. They're exotic and intriguing for beginners and a welcome respite for those who are tired of cheerleader aerobics with all its jumping up and down.

➤ Yoga

Due to its immense popularity, every variety of yoga is being offered today in clubs, and along with the variety of styles is a wide variance in quality. Some urban yoga classes are nothing more than power stretches with an Eastern flavor. Some of the more profound aspects of the mind-body-spirit integration have been shoved aside.

Still, you'll find a good class if you can find a yoga teacher who respects the tradition and teaches with sensitivity. You can choose from Hatha yoga, with its emphasis on breath and mind-body-spirit integration; Ivengar, with its emphasis on form and correct posture; Kripalu, with its inward focus and prolonged hold; and even Ashtanga, an aerobically paced sequence of asanas that stokes your fire.

10

Reclaim Your Inner Trainer

Many people think that they need a personal trainer to keep them motivated, yet the mere act of hiring someone else to help make you exercise immediately cuts away at any natural wisdom you have about what's good for your body. The trainer tells you what exercises to do, and you do them, whether you enjoy them or not. Eventually, you start skipping your appointments.

The way to get fit and stay fit is not to pay someone else to get you there. Rather, finding instinctual fitness involves discovering and reclaiming your own inner trainer. It's the most trustworthy voice you can listen to and the most reliable way to make instinctual fitness a self-fulfilling birthright.

The finest personal trainers that you can ever have are your own inspiration and intuition. With focused effort, your inspiration turns into perspiration. Like a trainer at a gym, your inspiration motivates you into action. Unlike that trainer, however, your inspiration motivates you into actions that your body craves and that you will enjoy—actions that will make you feel wonderful.

Your intuition comes from your deepest sense of self-worth, an honest watchdog of what's best for you. You've already learned a lot about how to tap into your intuition in chapter 6. Here, I'm going to offer you a few more tools to help you explore a particular kind of intuition, the kind that makes itself known during your dreams and most quiet moments and guides your largest efforts.

Developing your inspiration and intuition will provide endless payoffs.

They are always with you. They're free. And once you learn to tap into them, you will wonder how you ever got along without giving them your full attention. I'm going to teach you specific ways to cultivate your inspiration as well as help you tap even further into your intuition. With practice, these qualities will serve as your personal trainers, fitness buddies, coaches, and best friends, all in one.

GETTING INSPIRED

The word *inspiration* comes from the Latin "spiro," which means "filled with breath and life energy." Inspiration can prompt you to do things that you have never done before. Think of the young jock who falls in love and suddenly starts writing poems. Think of the older CEO who sits in his first wisdom circle with Native Americans and suddenly gives his money away.

Inspiration can make you move as you have never moved before. It can motivate you much more than any trainer yelling threats and perky remarks about feeling the burn. As you grow more attentive to the first stirrings of inspired sensation, you'll notice how your confidence builds, your courage swells, and your heart asks your backbone to accompany it boldly into new action.

Inspiration comes in a billion different ways. Racers, Strollers, Dancers, and Trekkers, however, use different muses to inspire them into action.

→ Racers: Inspired by Acts of Courage

Because your driving force requires frequent refueling, acts of courage—efficient, fast, results-oriented leadership—will inspire you most. Here are some examples of how you can use courageous acts to inspire intuitive fitness.

Competition. A turn-off for other movement types, competitive sports and recreational tournaments are complete and utter picnics for Racers. At least, they are for Racers who have learned to temper their confrontational and adversarial natures. If you still equate competition with combat, any sport can deteriorate into a belligerent power struggle. Learn to have fun, lighten up on other players, and share the authority so you can reap the most from competitive efforts.

Confidence games. Capitalize on your yen for leadership by playing games like paintball and war games in which you can act like a general. Your challenge with these games is to teach "subordinates" with true leadership and protection rather than simply growing drunk on power.

Skills training. You would make an excellent camp counselor, skills development coach, or ropes course trainer. Because you're magnanimous with your leadership skills, you have a natural instinct for inspiring others, especially those who look up to you or need your coaching.

Conditions that have an element of danger demand that you be strong-willed, but they also bring out your protective, nurturing qualities.

⊚ Strollers: Inspired by Acts of Comfort

Strollers love to spend time with family and friends in a relaxed, personal, and supportive atmosphere. Because you instinctively know how to create the most cozy surroundings, your biggest challenge is to overcome inertia and rouse yourself into action. When you want to inspire yourself into

---

GET OVER THAT HUMP

Of all of the movement personality types, Strollers sometimes have the toughest time hearing their inner trainer when it says "It's time to move." Inertia can be a very strong thing. That's why I'm offering the following psychological motivators to help you get through that initial "Oh, do I really have to do this now?" phase and move on to "Wow, this feels great. I'm glad I started moving."

Strollers often talk themselves out of moving by making up lame excuses. If you're a Stroller, you know all too well what I'm talking about.

For instance, many Strollers use the excuse, "I don't have any energy." Well, if you habitually tell yourself that you have no energy, it's time to get real and honest about it. If you have insufficient energy, exercise helps you generate more. The healthiest and best-looking form of stored energy is muscle glycogen, and you shore it up by moving your muscles. (Fat is the other form. You don't need more of that.) If you're really at a low ebb and physically spent, you can still benefit from doing some energy generators (see page 88).

Another common excuse is "I have no time." Moving really doesn't take much time. Instead of making a half-hour commitment, simply walk during lunch, park farther from your destination, use the stairs instead of the elevator, convert your coffee break into a movement break, and be honest about how much time you waste zoning out or doing not-so-healthy pastimes.

---

movement, make sure you work within your own time schedule and include other people.

You'll become even more inspired if you offer assistance to others. Here are some examples of activities that will comfort you while you become inspired to move.

Neighborhood sporting events. Arrange Little League games or soccer tournaments for children, friends, or co-workers. Just finding your way to the center of activity is a good idea for Strollers. Your natural inclination to extend your good will or volunteer your services will find you running the concession stand at local games or organizing T-shirt drives. Soon, friends will cajole you into picking up a racquet for a game of doubles or trying your turn at bat in a softball game.

Parties. Organize a tradition-bound gathering that benefits people you trust and love. Have an anniversary party, company picnic, or baby shower, but build some physical activity into it. Create a madcap scavenger hunt that involves everyone in canvassing the neighborhood. Or make sure the party has physical contests or lots of dancing. You could also gather friends for a charity fun-run to support a local cause or a national one, such as Race for the Cure.

Local recreation programs. Get involved with your local community parks and recreation agency. Start by taking a variety of classes—everything from beginner yoga to aqua aerobics. These organizations also need creative classes, outgoing instructors, and the support of people like you. You may very well find a class you like and become skilled at it, then find yourself in the next brochure, offering it with a new twist. Strollers are famous for becoming active by first sticking their toes in the water, then becoming indispensable to others and being coaxed into an active role. Enjoy the progression; it's your nature.

Dance classes. You're fortunate that interest in swing, lindy-hop, ballroom dancing and salsa are at an all-time high. Classes are available at health clubs, ballrooms, and nightclubs.

Group exercise. Finding friends and signing up for a fun aerobics class or other group class such as indoor cycling is a perfect outlet for Strollers.

✳ Dancers: Inspired by Acts of Beauty

Everyone admires glorious sunsets and snow-capped mountain ranges, but such awesome views serve as true sources of inspiration for Dancers. As quickly as you are inspired, however, you are also "de-inspired." Poor follow-through and the disapproval of others can crush these sudden inspirations, plunging you into the black hole of incomplete dreams that every Dancer keeps well-hidden.

Understand that although your inspirations are sometimes fleeting and superficial, you can integrate them more fully into your life by perceiving their essential attractive features. Your challenge is to temper your inspiration with insight and with the knowledge that what you have right now may just be enough. Here are some good activities that will inspire you with beauty.

Dance. Dancers are born to dance, and there's never been a better time for that. Classes are springing up all over in a national resurgence of folk dancing, ballroom, and swing. You can take advantage of the marriage of aesthetics and athleticism that dance provides to get a great workout.

Natural wonders. The natural beauty of the great outdoors will always seduce Dancers to move in a variety of ways. Because you bore easily with one routine, seasonal changes offer the variety that you require. Whether it's hiking through the wildflowers of spring or snowshoeing in winter, you draw your inspiration from the sights that surround you. Soak up the sights, sounds, and smells of nature. You will eventually take your love-of-nature–inspired fitness to new heights and challenge yourself with river rafting, rock climbing, horseback riding, sea kayaking, and mountain biking.

Spontaneous movement. Dancers give in to wild, spontaneous acts that may seem reckless to the other types, but their passion for experiencing life in these sudden bursts can keep them fit and happy. Because your imagination is ignited by the most ordinary acts, you can be inspired to move by the first song you hear on the radio or by the message on a billboard or bumper sticker. You tend to find meaning in almost everything and look for the beauty within. Relish the way it feels to move your body in new ways to random songs on the radio. Walk around and gesture gracefully as you "conduct" to the sounds of classical music.

Trekkers: Inspired by Acts of Intelligence

The right information is a significant motivator for Trekkers, who respond favorably to convincing data and statistics. You make change through small adjustments achieved with cautious strides. You don't drop routines suddenly but do so incrementally. Thoroughness and preparation take precedence over disorganization or illogical sudden starts.

Information alone is motivating for approximately 2 out of 10 people in my studies, not for the vast majority. That 20 percent is usually made up of Trekkers. You tend to analyze information and appreciate having all the facts in order to make a decision. That's why acts of high intelligence can inspire you to make the extraordinary commitment to fitness and movement. For inspiration, check "The Incredible Benefits of Getting Fit" or develop a personalized list. Also, start the following inspirational habits.

Daily log. Keep a written scorecard of the quantity and quality of your daily movement in an activity log. This will help you track your progress and translate your movement pursuits into tangible data that is easily analyzed. Moreover, the log will motivate you by its mere presence: You don't want the record to show that you are skipping out on life-affirming movement!

THE INCREDIBLE BENEFITS OF GETTING FIT

The following is a list of my favorite reasons to move, based upon 25 years of research and recently compiled in a groundbreaking manual, the *U.S. Surgeon General's Report on Physical Activity and Health*. Post this list where you can be nudged daily by its compelling evidence. Here's what movement can do for you.

- Increase overall energy and stamina
- Strengthen your heart and circulatory system and increase endurance
- Increase lung capacity, function, and volume
- Increase muscle strength and endurance
- Increase flexibility and mobility
- Maintain ideal body weight and improve body composition
- Improve metabolic functioning and the ability to burn fat for energy
- Lower the risk of sports and recreational injury
- Shorten postnatal recovery time for new mothers
- Increase sexual desire and confidence
- Reduce the likelihood of unhealthy habits such as smoking and poor diet
- Improve circulation
- Increase IQ in older people
- Enhance the ability to relax in stressful situations
- Lead to improved self-image and enhanced self-esteem

Personal progress charts. Actually chart your monthly progress on graph paper. Seeing a visual representation—whether it's expressed in minutes of movement per day, number of pounds lifted, walking speed, or whatever—will provide the objective feedback you need to keep pursuing fitness.

Health tests. Have your body fat, cholesterol levels, blood pressure, and other health indicators tested by a professional, then be tested again at regular intervals. The numbers alone will inspire you to improve.

Personal fitness tests. Find every chart, quiz, or test of your fitness, flexibility, biological age, and so forth that you can. Take the tests and see how you measure up. It's a powerful motivator for Trekkers to know that they are registering good scores.

Shared progress reports. Check out health clubs and community recreation

- Build optimism, psychological hardiness, and positivity
- Enhance creativity and problem-solving
- Uplift emotional spirits
- Provide the energy to explore new challenges, meaning, and purpose in life
- Provide the companionship of positive people who share belonging, intimacy, and friendship
- Lower the risk of premature death from cancer and cardiovascular disease
- Lower total cholesterol and raise good HDL cholesterol
- Reduce blood pressure
- Decrease the risk of osteoporosis, improving bone health
- Reduce insomnia and promote more restful sleep
- Increase blood flow, improving the condition of your skin
- Lower the risk of breast cancer
- Reduce the likelihood of premenstrual syndrome
- Reduce the risk of endometriosis, a primary cause of infertility
- Reduce by two-thirds the risk of type 2 (non-insulin-dependent) diabetes
- Reduce the need for insulin for type 1 (insulin-dependent) diabetes
- Ease leg spasms and improve the condition of varicose veins
- Reduce arthritis pain and help keep joints flexible
- Relieve irritable bowel, indigestion, constipation, and other gastric conditions

centers for seasonal contests of fitness participation and progress. A little bit of competition might be just the thing for Trekkers.

INTUITION FROM A HIGHER SOURCE

To listen more closely to your intuition, follow these pointers offered through the ages by three of the world's largest religions. If you don't believe in a higher power, the advice will still help you to motivate yourself. If you do believe in a higher power, however, the following will be all the more meaningful to you.

The Mahabharata. "Fully act, but do not be attached to the outcome," advised Krishna. From Hinduism's holy book, we learn that happiness comes from being aware of what is currently happening. As attachment increases, happiness dissipates. Intuitive fitness is not obsessed with obtaining results. "Results" are that which hasn't happened yet. When you move joyously in the present moment, you are not attached to the results. Discard the image of

LEARN FROM YOUR LIMITATIONS

Can you give yourself permission to have "greasy hair" or "protruding belly" days? Those are the times when you just want to stay in bed and pull the covers over your head, the days when you're in a slump and any exertion seems manic.

During those times, it will seem that everything you've learned and all the new tools you've acquired are failing you. On those days when no physical activity appeals to you, there's still a way to move your body comfortably. You can continue to work toward feeling light, energetic, and spontaneous despite coping with stonelike density.

First, you have to meet yourself exactly where you are. You simply knock gently on the door of your limitation, then breathe, rest, and be with it, without judgment. My yoga teacher, for example, can normally bend over and touch her forehead to her knees—but sometimes she can't. When those "sometimes" show up, she used to stretch, strain, and force her way to the maximum ideal point. Then she realized how she was damaging her muscles and ligaments and missing the whole point of yoga. The experience lies in coming up against the point of limitation, wherever it may happen to be that day.

what you are supposed to look like, and begin moving simply for the pure pleasure of it.

The Talmud. "You don't have to finish the work, but you must not desist from doing it." This phrase from the wise Jewish text tells us that we can use goals as guides, but we shouldn't become overwrought by them. Too unrealistic a goal will push you to overextend yourself, stretching too much and exhausting your reserves. When you realize that fitness is not about finishing, you intuitively stretch just the right amount—neither too little nor too much. You ignore the arbitrary quotas of exercise because you are reading your body, never desisting from the right amount of activity.

The Bible. In the creation story, God rested on the seventh day, and from then on, God requested that humans do the same. There's something delicious about the deep restorative rest that follows a massive, sustained physical effort. I've rock-climbed with friends for more than eight hours and then laughed myself silly with fatigue that night over beer and Mexican food. You sleep the sleep

Allow that limitation to teach you something about yourself: how much stress you've been living with lately, how your diet has been, how hungover you feel, how you've been more sedentary than usual, how you haven't stretched in a while, and so on. You will get a physical readout from your inner voice while you hang out in that tough spot.

Second, you have to let go of any criticism and judgment about those limits and uncomfortable conditions. If you ignore this limitation and power over it, going for some memory of former greatness, your ego, not your sensory awareness, will be in charge of your workout. You'll bypass the rich feedback that you could be getting.

Third, you have to do it more easily and more gently than you've ever let yourself move or exercise before. Continue to practice your breathwork, even though your breathing will seem shallow and labored. Do your biorhythmic movements for dawn, daytime, and dusk, even though they may seem so curtailed that you wonder if it's worth the effort. It is.

Take a lesson from aikido masters and don't confront your limits head-on, feeding in your own frustration and pent-up explosive energy. Focus on practice, not mastery, and do it with the ease that the best Eastern meditative teachers call quiet vitality.

of the grateful dead on a night like that, and although your body reminds you of your excesses the next day, the smile creeps back because rest never felt so good.

When you allow yourself to rest, you give your muscles a chance to heal and your mind a chance to reboot. Deep rest also brings you more in touch with your inner stirrings. After taking a day off, you'll not only be inspired, your instincts will be strongly nudging you in the right direction.

LET YOUR DREAMS BRING INTUITION

Did you ever notice how well you move when you're dreaming? There is nothing like a little quiet REM time to make believe that you've mastered the most outrageous physical skills. You can float down stairs, waltz across ballrooms, and ride bareback.

In my dreams, I rise to a challenge like Wonder Woman, rescuing jumbo jets careening out of control. Not only do I suddenly understand the mechanics of aeronautics, but my body knows what to do.

The words of psychophysiologist Stephen LaBerge, author of *Lucid Dreaming* and *Exploring the World of Lucid Dreaming*, shed light on this dreamy realm and the magical body you occupy in it. In a lucid dream, you have a vivid awareness that you are actually in the middle of a dream. With this awareness, you can direct the outcome, substitute people or actions, and reinvent the circumstances.

This conscious act of directing and manipulating can leave you feeling oddly in charge of skills that would take years to develop. Not only do you have a sense of being gifted with physical mastery, you're also aware of creating your reality. At the onset of a few of my own dreams, I've even appeared with a top hat and cane, like a vaudeville master of ceremonies, and said to an invisible audience, "We interrupt this dream to make a few last-minute substitutions."

Dreams hold a magical value for various aspects of our waking states. Their images, feelings, and impressions not only help us clarify and enact specific intentions, they also help us make the dreams a reality. Just what is the impact on the physical body when you master a movement skill in a dream? Is learning taking place? Yes. Body and mind are two aspects of the same reality.

Besides helping us learn new skills, dreams also allow us to explore past experiences that may be keeping us from being fit today. Through dreams, I've been able to wind my way through densely fogged-over material such as my mother's countless hospitalizations, my brother's hostility, and my father's

REAL-LIFE INSTINCTS

Sometimes, to be better trainers, "we too have to let go and remember the true meaning of fitness. It is about having the energy to embrace the challenges of life, not simply to run for 30 minutes on a treadmill. It is a fusion of mind and body. It happens anytime, anywhere—even in the jungle," says Dora Zall, a Boston-based fitness trainer who discovered a fitness adventure far from her gym, in the jungles of Ecuador.

aloofness. In doing so, I've been able to free up a livelier, more authentic self. As a result, I have a profound respect for my body's ability to unfold early life dramas so that I can form new patterns of being with family and friends. It's as if my body plays out a scene so my courage, trust, and lively spirit can be liberated.

Once we travel with increasing ease and frequency between conscious and unconscious states, we note that the distance between the two points on this well-trodden pathway keeps growing shorter. The conscious and unconscious realms begin to have more identical characteristics. Intuition, synchronicity, the perfect timing of unexpected events—they all show up in both worlds whenever needed, whenever anticipated. Just as the physicist discovered that subatomic particles tend to appear where you expect to take a picture of them, our realities tend to emerge based on our intentions. Reality itself becomes a fluid medium, its boundaries nothing more than an impulse or potential that continually gives rise to the other levels of consciousness.

When you dream, you're doing choreography. Just like Fred Astaire in the old movie *Holiday Inn*, you have the freedom to experience yourself in extraordinary states. In the dream state, your body knows what to do. When you awaken, it's really your mind that won't allow you to duplicate the experience.

I've observed this phenomenon many times in operating rooms. When a patient is alert before surgery, she may move stiffly and slowly, guarding an injury or telling you that she is rather inflexible, that she can't bend too far or lift her leg behind her. She copes with all sorts of physical limitations. Once anesthetized, however, her mind lets go of its rigid control, and her body flops like a fish out of water. Limbs that were stiff are easily moved into wide stretches.

As you can see, tapping into your dreams can bring you wonderful, intuitive results, teaching you more about your waking body. Here's how to access your intuitive dream state.

- Recall your dreams in the very early waking moments before you get out of bed.
- Scan your body for any physical sensations that the dreams may have aroused.
- Look for new confidence in your physical capabilities.
- Listen to your inner voice about the dream's messages. Retain what's useful; forget the rest.
- Allow those select dream messages to serve as gentle guides in your physical actions throughout the day. If your dream involved some activity that you either observed or participated in, for example, find a way to do that activity during your waking life.

LEARN TO SEE IN THE DARK

No matter what your movement type—Racer, Stroller, Dancer, or Trekker—you must venture into new territory before you start to discover the keys to natural fitness. Like many intrepid explorers, you won't always have sufficient information to make the journey comfortable. That's why your intuitive skills must be honed in order to boldly go into the unknown, relying only on your gut instincts.

At first, you may feel that you desperately need someone to tell you what to do. That simply means that you must hang out in the unknown for a while, until it becomes comfortable. Then the answers will come to you.

Hanging out in the unknown means that you have to first "uncurse the darkness." You have to grow more accepting of ambiguities and uncertainties and not worry so much about not being in control. Think of some of the most exhilarating or physically challenging events in your life. You experienced them because you didn't know enough to prevent them from occurring, right? This is often how we are shoved along to take our first steps, whether it's getting off the wrong chair lift or discovering that the dude ranch vacation is more of a working cattle drive. If you can let go and trust the universe, you'll enjoy the ride a lot more. Be humble. Lose your footing. Grow weak and giddy with "I don't know." Intuition will follow like a cooling thunderstorm after unbearable humidity.

11

Find Your Hidden Motivation

Your body wants to move. Perhaps you can feel it. Those are the urgings of your fitness instinct—your seventh sense—at work. Now that you're tapped into your movement instinct and your natural movement personality—which takes its cues from your seventh sense—as well as armed with enjoyable new ways to move, you're almost ready to embark on a lifetime of successful fitness.

I say "almost" because you have one final step to go. To start moving and stay moving, you must unleash your endless supply of natural motivation.

Motivation is an inner drive that compels you to behave in a certain way. Motivation can turn lethargy into energy. It can inspire you to move as you have never moved before. I'm going to teach you one of life's best-kept secrets: how to find this motivation and have it on hand at all times.

Many of us are guilty of thinking that motivation is something that comes and goes, something that we get by chance or maybe by luck, when the heavenly muses decide to give us a dose. Perhaps we base this belief on the way motivation seems to dry up when we're faced with a less-than-desirable task. The truth is, however, that motivation never leaves you. It's there all the time. You simply may be directing it to a temporary diversion. Let me explain.

Instead of thinking of motivation as something that comes and goes upon its own whim, imagine it as a constant in your life. You are always motivated to do something, but whether it fits your present picture of acceptable acts is another story.

For instance, let's say that you've undertaken a new exercise routine, and your motivation to pursue it is at an all-time high. Then your best friend comes in from out of town and can only meet you at the airport in the morning—right in the middle of your committed exercise hour. You skip your session and have a great reunion. What happened to your motivation? Did it wane in the face of a social get-together? Are you a slouch beyond redemption?

No, your motivation simply moved. You were more motivated to reconnect with an old pal than to take one more run around the block. And that's my point: You're always motivated to do something, because generally, we are always doing something, even if it's resting.

Another example: You're in your car, and you reach for your wallet to pull out some cash. A dollar bill flies out the window at a busy intersection. Do you stop the car to go chase it? If traffic is pretty busy, maybe not. What if it were $100? Or $500? Suddenly, the idea of sprinting across a few lanes of speeding traffic seems worth it.

What shifts is the value, seriousness, or priority that we assign to each act.

You are always motivated to move. The problem is, sometimes your natural motivation is blocked by destructive thoughts, many of them taught to us by well-meaning fitness professionals. Such destructive tactics, such as forcing yourself to work out simply to attain a thinner, shapelier body, camouflage your natural motivation.

Your natural motivation to move also may compete with your motivation to eat, sleep, and socialize. Sometimes, those other callings should take precedence over exercise, and sometimes they shouldn't. Learning to know the difference involves tapping fully into your fitness instinct and in following my four steps to discovering fitness motivation.

OFFER YOURSELF INTRINSIC REWARDS

When I worked in community mental health centers, the nurses and doctors practiced aversion therapy, a harsh method of "motivating" alcoholics to stop drinking. They tried to train an alcoholic's mind and body to be repelled by the smell of the very stuff he craved. They placed the unfortunate drinker in a small, windowless room filled with open bottles of booze so the scent of liquor was thick. Then they injected him with a chemical that induced severe gagging and vomiting. There the poor patient sat, a stainless-steel bowl in his lap, heaving up his guts.

Associating the smell of the liquor with vomiting may seem like the height of inhuman conditioning, but it worked for about 20 percent of those treated. Many patients did return to drinking, however, and eventually, aversion therapy met its demise.

Many of us still carry around this kind of cruel, ineffective "motivational" tool. Have you ever posted a picture of yourself during your chubbier days near the fridge? Have you ever called yourself a fat pig to motivate yourself through an aerobics session?

Don't feel guilty if you have. It doesn't mean that you have a warped mind. You probably got these ideas from the gym or from some magazines.

Negative motivation isn't without its usefulness. Many of us experience it in our everyday lives. It is what you feel when you go on a diet because you just spent a Saturday trying on clothes in the store, and nothing seemed to fit. It's what my child felt when she stopped sucking her thumb to avoid the ridicule at school.

Yet, if you've tried negative motivation before, you've probably found that it doesn't work for long. If the event that originally triggered the action starts to fade from memory, there will not be enough fuel to keep your wheels in motion.

Take the case of the son of one of my cardiac patients. Dave, a 45-year-old accountant, started exercising when his father had a heart attack. The push behind his desire to exercise arose from a negative source—fear of heart disease and death. After a few weeks, though, Dave dropped out of his routine because his father got better. Dave just wasn't as scared anymore. The fact that his dad continued in a successful phase of exercise maintenance and cardiac rehabilitation didn't seem to motivate Dave.

Although it may be useful in the beginning, negative motivation is often not enough impetus to keep you going for a lifetime commitment. Is there a better way? Of course. According to research on adherence, incentive therapy produces far more preferable and lasting outcomes.

Sports psychologists recommend that people switch from negative motivation to positive motivation as soon as possible in order to stick to their commitments. This means rewarding yourself with something pleasurable after you accomplish a particular positive behavior. An example of this would be parents who reward a teenager with the keys to the family car once she improves her grades. You could take yourself on a shopping spree after your first trip to the gym.

Positive motivation is self-reinforcing because it allows you to continue an action for the rewards and benefits. They become the drive. Even positive motivation, however, must evolve from external rewards into intrinsic rewards in order to be sustaining.

What do I mean by external and intrinsic? External rewards are things you use to prod yourself along, to force yourself to move. They simply don't originate from deep within your body, mind, and soul.

Yes, rewarding yourself with things such as a gourmet dinner, new clothes, or a long weekend is pleasurable, and yes, it can work. It's nowhere near as effective, though, as intrinsic rewards, the ones that come from deep within. Examples: The stress relief and endorphin boost that you get from a quick stroll around the block on a beautiful day. The pain relief and emotional oneness that you find during and after a yoga class. The relief you feel as the tension drains out of your neck and back when you get up from your desk, walk around, and stretch.

When you are motivated intrinsically, you no longer prod yourself to move. You no longer hold a carrot in front of your nose. Rather, you move for the sheer feeling of moving. You move because you enjoy it.

Jonathan Robinson, Ph.D., director of the Michigan Center for Preventive Medicine in Lansing, has been challenging the wisdom of using behavior modification rewards to promote health. From the classroom to the workplace, he and other researchers have found that external rewards, while they may help with some short-term change in attitude, fail to prompt lasting changes. In fact, Alfie Kohn, author of *Punished by Rewards: The Trouble with Gold Stars, Incentive Plans, A's, Praise, and Other Bribes*, says that there is quite a bit of evidence that such rewards may even inhibit learning, productivity, and creativity.

You know that you've reached the golden landscape of intrinsic rewards or intuitive motivation when you feel joy and flow in your activity—when you can experience what University of Chicago researcher Mihaly Csikszentmihalyi, Ph.D., calls a combination of playfulness and discipline. Without these joyful attributes, all the external rewards in the world wouldn't be enough to motivate your efforts into new territories.

With intrinsic rewards, you experience creativity. You sense the exhilaration of peak performance. You feel the afterglow of physical activity. All of that serves as its own reward.

If you've spent years forcing yourself to move—and failing—you may not be able to switch your focus overnight. Be patient. Break your journey into small steps.

Move quickly away from negative motivation. Stop saying, "I'm sick and tired of looking this way. I'm going to work out until I drop from exhaustion."

Visit short-term external rewards. "After this workout, I deserve a day at the mall and lobster for two."

Arrive and stay with intrinsic rewards. "I get something from exercise that I just can't explain, but it's enough to keep me coming back for more."

MOVE TODAY, NOT TOMORROW

Too often, well-meaning career, time-management, and lifestyle counselors have asked us to make lists. You know what I mean: You generally are told to prioritize what you feel should be important in your life and write down short-term and long-term goals to help you keep those priorities front and center. You then establish a contract with yourself that goes something like "I will achieve (fill in the blank) by (fill in a date.)"

Such goal setting has served countless people. For many, however, it's been only a temporary fix. In my surveys of goal setting, I've found that this method works for only 2 out of 10 people. What happens to the other 8? Chances are, many of you fall into that group.

Conventional goal-setting techniques have many pitfalls. First of all, they don't last. Have you ever written down a goal, then posted it in a calendar or log or maybe on the refrigerator door? What happens after one week? Two weeks? In surveys, I found that after about 10 days, most people don't even see the note on the refrigerator.

Goal setting fades from your mind because it was never really locked into your imagination in the first place. Einstein said that an imagination is a far greater asset than a mind. For the most part, goal setting does not come from deep within you, since you usually put it into practice like a learned assignment rather than a passionate pursuit.

Second, these techniques work against your natural instincts. They make you focus on the goal, not the path. When you're continually focused on the whole enormous task ahead of you, you can quickly become overwhelmed and demoralized, even if you break it down into short-term steps such as getting to the gym three times a week. Your mind knows the bigger picture and isn't fooled by the shortened version. Lisa Stephen says in her book *Willpower* that the distance between where you are now and where you want to be can seem like the distance from here to another galaxy.

Third, this kind of goal setting reinforces what's wrong with you. It never allows you to reframe yourself as the person you want to be. Again, the focus remains on the end picture—the "you" who is thinner or richer or whatever.

Here's a much better way. Instead of saying, "Someday, I want to be (fill in the blank)," state your goal in the present and make the personal transformation right now. It's the difference between saying, "I'm going on a diet," and saying, "I eat healthy, well-balanced, nutritious foods that manage my desired weight naturally." See the difference? The former suspends an illusory reality before you; the latter places you firmly in that reality right now.

Because it is a way of describing your future and not your present, goal setting has the deactivating, built-in flaw of shifting the focus to an endpoint. When we are focused on the outcome, we tend to lift out of the present moment.

Even if we imagine the desired end result as a mental tractor beam pulling us toward it, the most successful lifestyle changes occur when the lion's share of attention is fixed on the process rather than the destination. Learning to live with the day-to-day process in present-time awareness is the real key to successfully transforming your life. In fact, this shift is so extraordinary in its transformative quality that it allows you to leave the world of incremental steps and enter a life of fundamental, core-level change.

You're able to make a quantum leap because you've taken the rigidity out of how you view the achievement of goals. You've also taken the rigidity out of how you live. Similar to what's happened to global corporations in the last decade, you become lean and agile in your functioning. Ten-year plans are a joke in the business world, a leftover from an age of bureaucratic centralization. The pace of the world today insists on flexibility, creativity, responsiveness, and multidimensional processing. It thrives on freshness, irreverence, and bucking the system.

I've spoken with hundreds of people who made dramatic lifestyle turnarounds, and not one attributed the changes to conventional goal-setting techniques. In fact, I've become such an advocate of present-time awareness that I believe the older techniques are actually detrimental to the 8 out of 10 who continue to struggle with them.

When your health and fitness depend on achieving a long-term, step-by-step goal, you're merely presiding over the orderly march toward death. You're never all right, right now. Life isn't lived now, it's postponed until the time "when you're fit." The goal is always out there—something that can only be achieved by inching somewhere else. By dropping it, you energize yourself internally and move more harmoniously. Paradoxically, you can enjoy the pauses between the actions rather than feeling guilty about them.

To practice present-time awareness, or mindfulness, you have to give your attention to process. You can't just think abstractly about "present time" or give yourself a command to get in the present. It doesn't work that way. Instead, you throw the switch to present time by gliding along your breath, focusing on a mantra or words of special meaning. The magic of mantra-paired-with-breath will escort you to present time. Here are some to try.

When you're overloaded with too much to do: Inhale while you think, "With every breath, I connect to my source." Exhale while you think, "From here, I have plenty of time to do all I can."

When you're upset by circumstances beyond your control: Inhale while you think, "I breathe in the world around me." Exhale while you think, "I breathe out how I choose to experience the world."

When you want to return to present-time awareness: Cultivate a special sound of your own choice, such as the Sanskrit words for breath, *Sa* and *Hahm*. Inhale, then say "Sa" or "Hahm" as you breathe out. It should sound like a melodious hum: "Saaaaaaa" or "Hahmmmmmmmmmm."

You can also use the words *Ma* and *Pa* to symbolize your connection with Mother Earth and Father Time.

AIM FOR AN IN-YOUR-BODY EXPERIENCE

You're breathing heavily and sweating like crazy. Your heart rate is flying. Your muscles are feeling the burn. Yet nobody is home. I have interviewed more than 100 instructors who admitted that they can teach an entire aerobics class and somehow not be present. They feel as if they have checked out of their bodies. I have interviewed women and men who say that they just "get through" exercise by checking out and thinking about something else because it is so boring. I was amazed at a couple of disclosures in these conversations:

one, that so many people routinely disembody in order to do their workouts, and two, that so many people are completely adept at it.

When you need to distract yourself and mentally check out in order to move, you're not staying present. This chips away at your motivation.

In chapter 6, I introduced you to the notion of embodiment, that is, how to always have a sense of the state of your physical being. Given its importance, I want to elaborate on its causes and broaden its meaning and impact.

How and why we leave our bodies is a topic that's beyond the scope of this book. Still, I believe that we live with many influencing factors—family dysfunction, abusive relationships, violence, pornography, and harassment. Any of them can push you into a checked-out, unaware, shut-down, disembodied state.

BREAK OLD HABITS FOR GOOD

Even the most willful characters could use some help breaking old habits now and then. For the most part, however, we're far too critical of ourselves in declaring our number of poor habits. I find that the only really poor habit that people need to break is making up lame excuses when it comes to fitness. I offer this last-ditch advice in case you need to unlock one more motivational force within you.

When it comes to excuse busting, it helps to regard the universe in its polarized aspect. For everything that exists, its opposite also exists. Female-male. Night-day. All-nothing. Quantum mechanics teaches us not only that the universe is a field of infinite possibilities, with multiplicity and chaos running the show, but also that within that pattern, dichotomous structures also exist. The Chinese call it yin-yang, and the Greeks considered it a law of nature. For every shining trait that we like to show, we probably have a weakness that we don't like to admit lurking in the shadows.

I believe that for every excuse, there is an excuse buster—perfectly matched pairs, two ends of the same continuum. We already have a good idea of how skilled we are at making excuses, so for a minute or two, let's practice creating excuse busters.

Excuse: I'm too tired to do anything.
Excuse buster: I get energy when I take a walk.

Excuse: I'm out of time.
Excuse buster: Time passes no matter what I do—if I'm still or if I'm moving. So I'm moving in creative ways right now.

If you have deep issues with your body—you hate the way it looks or you think it's "dirty"—you must put those issues aside before you can uncover your natural motivation. That may take counseling, or it may take only a new mindset.

Bodies come in all shapes and sizes. Acknowledging that yours is unique is the first step toward recognizing its beauty. Learning to stay present in your body and not becoming disembodied through shame or self-disgust is an act of loving kindness. The more generous you are in appreciating your body, the more your natural, unique beauty is available for others to see as well.

Did you ever hear a small child call his grandma the most beautiful woman in the world? The beauty that the child sees is alive in the love and light that emanates from the elderly grandmother as she gazes at her grandchild. Appre-

---

Excuse: I get too bored when I exercise.
Excuse buster: Boredom comes from stagnancy. Movement shakes it off. Now you fill in the blanks.

An excuse I've used in the past: _____.
Excuse buster: _____.

Now, you're probably wondering how you'll know when an excuse is really valid. For instance, if you have the flu and skip exercising because you're too tired, that's a real excuse. Believe me, you'll know. When your excuse rings hollow, it doesn't make the phone ring deep inside you. Your body-scam detector will sound its full alarm.

The next time you find yourself making an excuse not to move, take yourself through the following five steps.

H: Make sure your *heart* is really in it. Sincerity is crucial.
A: Become fully *aware* of the moment at which the old habit or excuse appeared.
B: *Break* the pattern. Take a deep *breath*, focus, and act on the alternative.
I: *Immerse* yourself in positive affirmations. State the change you want in the present tense: "I am calm and centered and ready to move."
T: *Train* yourself to do this over and over. Be kind to yourself. Don't expect to get it right each time—after all, you're in training.

ciation is the gateway to seeing real beauty. Let it open your lens and change how you view your own body.

As a student of world religion, I have sought out the commonalities that weave through diverse spiritual traditions, including Sufism, Judaism, Christianity, Islam, Buddhism, Hinduism, and various Native American, Aboriginal, and North African belief systems. Although some threads can be woven through religious traditions with similar origins, such as Judaism, Christianity, and Islam, I am always awestruck at the widely divergent ways in which cosmologies are constructed by various tribes of this human family. We are more different than I thought.

There is only one thread, one commonality, and it is indisputable: We all have bodies. It is the only obvious link among people with differing gods, creation stories, values, customs, mythologies, preferences, and more. The body stands out as the living testament to spirit made manifest in each of us, and as such, it should be held most sacred. Not just its pristine and cleansed appearance, but all the ooze and decay and abundant flesh as well. For me, the body, experienced through the senses, including the sixth sense of intuition and the seventh sense of intuitive movement, is how we know the Divine. What the body informs us and feels for us is how we experience Goddess/God.

Intuitive motivation starts with being in your body. You have to occupy it more fully than you ever have. You can generate your own imagery to accomplish this easily. Start with taking some deep breaths and focusing inward. Progress to enjoying the feeling of movement. Feel your legs move. Feel air as it comes in and out of your nose or mouth. Really feel the movement.

If you have trouble doing this, try the walking meditation or visualizations described in chapter 5. They will help you get in touch with your body in a healthy way.

TAP INTO YOUR CORE DESIRE

Offering yourself positive, intrinsic rewards is a start. Thinking in the present and enjoying the process rather than the goal is also great. To truly have motivation by your side 24 hours a day, seven days a week, however, you must tap into your core desire.

I've seen hundreds of people harness their natural movement instinct and drive for success with this brilliant path toward self-renewal and continuous motivation.

Some of my thinking on core desire was inspired by Jack Zufelt, named

America's great motivator by *Who's Who*. Raised on a Navajo Indian reservation in Arizona, he was the only Anglo-American in his high school class. Until the age of 14, his family had no television or telephone. The unlikely mix of his upbringing, his cultural legacy, and his experience in training gave him a startling new perspective on the origins of motivation.

Zufelt agrees with me that traditional goal setting for health and fitness is a waste of time for most people. He says, "If you follow the principles and teachings of most training instructors, I have found they don't work as everyone expects them to. The motivation lasts only a few days. What works is the ability to clearly define our core desires."

Core desires are the genuine, clearly defined wants that make you willing to put forth any effort necessary to make those desires a reality, even when it means overcoming staggering odds. Core desire is not just a wish or a dream. It is derived from the deepest center of your being. Nothing can stop it.

You have already experienced the power of your core desire at some point in your life. It was there during those times when you needed to accomplish something in such a hurry that it felt as if you stopped time in order to pull it off. Because they tap a higher source, core desires contain the power to move mountains. You usually have one working in a predominant way at any given time. Moreover, core desires shift on you. One will take center stage while the others recede, and then they switch again at different times of your life.

When I ask people what they really want, they often draw a blank. Since you may not be able to clearly feel what your core desire is, I've developed a little story and related matching game that will help you identify it. You can also look at the core desires of your friends and family and see what you can do to support their motivational inner fires as well.

Read through the following story. Have paper and a pencil handy, because you may want to jot down a few instant reactions to each segment of the story as you read it. First impressions are most important, though, so try not to over-analyze or ponder each case.

> *You were on a pleasure cruise in the South Pacific when a sudden hurricane and tidal wave overturned the vessel, washing you up on a tiny, desolate island. Right next to you is another island. When you scan it, you can tell that something on that island is definitely worth the effort that it would take to get there. But what an effort! The two tiny islands are separated by shark-infested waters, a real hazard to your survival.*

These sharks are stuporously slow, however, and you could outswim them, but not without great exertion.

Now, the question is, what is on that other island that makes you want to get there so badly? Below I've listed six different scenarios; read through them and pick the one that would make you put out the effort to cross those dangerous waters. Listen with your heart. Go with what's truest for you, with no judgment, no right or wrong.

Scenario 1. There are a few other survivors, all with smiles and beckoning waves, imploring you to join them. They look warm and inviting, and you're feeling very lonely.

Scenario 2. You spot a treasure chest overflowing with glittering riches. There's even a craft there that you could probably jury-rig to brave the ocean with the treasure chest.

Scenario 3. Your own island is a desolate, barren, bleak pile of sand, while the other is a beautiful tropical paradise with gloriously colored foliage, fruits, waterfalls, and rainbows. You're happy just gazing at it, so imagine what it would be like to live there.

Scenario 4. A group of natives inhabits that island. They look friendly but extremely naive and rather superstitious. With your wits and drive, you could create quite a kingdom for yourself, choose your mate, and rule in comfort and power.

Scenario 5. You see fascinating ruins of a lost civilization on the island that are eerily similar to the tales of Atlantis. You're moved by the magic and power of the vast knowledge of its one-time inhabitants and want to explore it in depth.

Scenario 6. You're not alone after all. A few survivors made it to your island, but they're turning it into a lawless, savage Club Med from Hell. You notice that the survivors on the other island are cooperating peaceably and organizing a community with order and harmony.

Now let's see what struck your fancy. Remember, you have many of these core desires circulating within your personality and psyche, but only one plays a dominant role. Once you know that core desire, you can attach your motivational drive to a customized goal. This will fuel your day-to-day actions better than anything I know.

Scenario 1. Your core desire is social. You have a desire for belonging and need emotional and physical contact with other people. Keep your schedule spontaneous and open to change. Since distractions can easily derail your efforts, try to stay focused.

The buddy system works best to help you stay motivated to move. Look for social groups, classes, ski trips, Sierra Club walks, dance classes, drumming circles, line dancing, inline skating with friends, and hiking and recreational groups.

Scenario 2. Your core desire is economic. You are motivated by monetary rewards and need to get the most out of every move, often carrying out multiple tasks at once to save time. Combine fitness with errands such as a run to an ATM or the dry cleaner. Walk to work. Circuit-train to combine cardiovascular and weight training.

Scenario 3. Your core desire is aesthetic. You're motivated by beauty and appealing environments. Your schedule should be well-organized, with sufficient blocks of time to escape to your inner peaceful state of mind. Move in beautiful settings. Build a fitness wardrobe of colors and textures that you love to wear. Create a movement room in your home: Paint the walls and decorate it in the most harmonious colors and designs. Go on nature hikes, cycle outdoors, or try jazz or expressive dance, improvisational theater, stretching, yoga, and body sculpting.

Scenario 4. Your core desire is political. You're motivated by a desire for authority and power. You need to set your schedule "in stone," or else a dozen urgent demands will take precedence. Try fast-paced aerobics classes, running, speedwalking, intense workouts with intermittent breaks, Spinning classes, competitive sports, race training, and triathlons.

Scenario 5. Your core desire is theoretical. You're motivated by a desire for knowledge. Beware of procrastination in favor of sedentary activities. Try body building, orienteering (trail reading), and walking tours. You'll enjoy cardiovascular machines set up for reading or watching the evening news, PBS, or the Discovery Channel. Use headphones during your walks so that you can listen to books on tape.

Scenario 6. Your core desire is methodical. You want rules, order, and harmony. Keep your schedule consistently timed and self-contained. Solo activities are just fine for you. The challenge is to build in flexibility and not become too obsessive about your chosen routine. Your best movement activities have a wide-open range. You will excel in anything that requires consistent application of training principles. Weight training, sports skill development, ballroom dance, ballet, gymnastics, horseback riding, and rock climbing are good choices.

chapter *12*

Quick Fixes: Let Your Instincts Guide You

We all have guilty desires. All of us. No matter how much we try to accept our bodies, our lives, and ourselves for what they are—no matter how well we tap into our fitness instincts—we sometimes can't help being tempted by quick fixes or shortcuts. You know the ones. The ad for the diet program that promises "one week to a perfect body." The cream we see in the store that promises to "abolish cellulite." The supplement that says it will "stop aging" or "eliminate joint pain."

Yes, we're tempted. And we're guilty. But you really can't blame us. With all the images we see every day on magazine covers, on television, in movies, on billboards—just about everywhere—of thin, young, "perfect" women and men, we can't help wanting to look just like them. While movement and healthful eating may help us look better, it will never make us look like supermodels. Thus, we turn to wishful thinking.

Before you close this book and go happily on your journey to instinctual fitness, I want to have a frank, pro-and-con discussion of these guilty desires, the almost naughty pleasure we feel when we think that just maybe, we can get something for nothing. No, I'm not abandoning my original premise. I am more committed than ever to achieving health and fitness through natural means. But I'm a reasonable purist, not a fanatic. There is nothing wrong with wondering if certain artificial tools are actually helpful in the quest—and that wondering starts to really peak about the time that you stride through your thirties and into your midforties and fifties, when you question adrenaline aerobics and sign up for your first mind-body stretch class.

That is also the time when you begin to wonder about plastic surgery and diet pills to counter that ever-increasing midlife spread. You start to ask questions you never asked before (and never thought you would): "Is liposuction really all that bad?" "Do body wraps work on cellulite?" "Can herbs help me lose weight?" "Will this pill turn me into a Roman Love God?"

The truth is that everyone who is interested in fitness is also interested in maintaining a certain vigor and youthfulness. After a while, the distinction blurs between wanting to feel youthful and seeking perfection. Next, you're demanding a pill to undo baldness, one to make you sexy, another to let you sleep, and another to help you remember which pills to take.

QUICK FIXES THAT WORK—OR DON'T

If you believe that menopause is a disease that requires drug management, that the golden years should be altered with cosmetic surgery, that a great sex life is available in a pill, and that you can never be too thin or too tight, you are emotionally vulnerable to the sales pitch of every con artist in the new health age. Therefore, I remind you to keep cultivating your still point. The quest for the perfect appearance is an insidious little demon in our culture. Take your time with this chapter and consider both the upside and downside of each of the following. Address the issue of self-enhancement honestly. Without that opportunity, any healthy desire can turn into a harmful obsession.

Here's an A-to-Z list of some natural and many not-so-natural ways to look and feel younger, thinner, and more energetic. Surprise: Many earn my full stamp of approval. As for most of the others, I recommend banishing them from your life.

➤ Amino Acids

The basic building blocks of all protein, amino acids are critical for cell renewal, growth, and sustaining life. Weight lifters swear by them, but their use remains controversial, and the risks of oversupplementation when taken alone or in combination have prompted warnings from many nutrition experts. Nevertheless, research on amino acids may just alter our intakes in the future. For now, your best sources of amino acids are high-quality animal products such as eggs, milk, and lean poultry, fish, and meat. Vegetarians can stock up on whole grains, seeds, and nuts to get their minimum requirements. Here's a look at what these nutrients may do.

- *Arginine* helps control blood pressure and may be vital for male sexual function.
- *Carnitine* is proving to be useful for fat metabolism.
- *Choline* is important for the functioning of neurotransmitters and other brain chemicals.
- *Glutamine* is recognized as a treatment for anxiety, helps to promote sleep and relaxation, reduces sugar cravings, and is beneficial in drug rehabilitation therapy.
- *Tryptophan* is an important precursor to serotonin in the brain, aids sleep and relaxation, and may help ease depression.
- *Tyrosine* is vital in dealing with stress and is good for the skin and thyroid gland.

➤ Aromatherapy

A small investment that reaps sweet scent-sations, aromatherapy is the simplest alternative health remedy. I like it because it helps you get to your still point, which may help you calm down and let go of your unrealistic expectations.

Thousands of years old, aromatherapy is the art and science of inducing moods with specific smells. These distinct odors affect the olfactory passages and send messages along your nerves to your brain, transforming stress or stimulating healing. The scents take you from relaxed to energized and from reflective to sensual.

Essential oils also can have antiseptic or anti-inflammatory qualities and can even help with respiratory congestion. Many are ideal massage oils because they are natural lubricants. Experiment with a few drops of essential oil over a heated bowl or candle and note its effect on your mind and body. Here's a list of some scents and their beneficial effects. (Never take an essential oil internally; they are very strong and can be toxic if ingested.)

- *Lavender* calms.
- *Eucalyptus* opens respiration.
- *Rose* sweetens.
- *Lemon* detoxifies.

- *Sage* clears and grounds.
- *Peppermint* soothes.
- *Chamomile* lifts mood.
- *Rosemary* eases muscle tension.
- *Juniper* lifts fatigue.

➤ Body Image Acceptance

My teacher in body image and size acceptance is Pat Lyons, R.N., founder of Connections, Women's Health Consulting Network and co-author of *Great Shape*. She taught me that fat prejudice is the last safe prejudice, fueling body shame. "Girls and women are preoccupied with the size of their thighs rather than the size of their dreams. Chronic dieting, frenetic exercise, and eating disorders are frighteningly commonplace, and the real public health disaster—the cardiac damage that resulted from a diet pill frenzy—has mysteriously disappeared under the carpet, while a new production pipeline of pills goes on," Lyons says. She is calling for a national campaign, Free at Last: The Women's Body Sovereignty Project, and asks you to consider some simple actions.

- Stop making comments about weight—yours or other people's—especially in front of children or teens.
- Educate yourself about healthy alternatives to dieting and weight-loss–focused medical care.
- Take time to nurture and appreciate your body. To get some help on body image acceptance, read books, join a support circle, attend workshops, and call Lyons. To join her national efforts with community speakouts, workshops, and professional training, send e-mail to plyons@earthlink.net.

➤ Cellulite Creams and Machines

There are still health experts who argue that there is no such thing as cellulite, but most women know better. Baruch Jacobs, M.D., is a Miami-area plastic surgeon who doesn't mind using the word *cellulite*. He knows that when fat cells grow larger, the subcutaneous connective tissue compresses and hardens, making blood circulation more difficult and leading to increased tension on the underlying skin. The bumpy, irregular appearance is most common on the thighs, hips, buttocks, and belly. Call it cellulite or call it "regular" fat—most women would grant a Nobel prize to the chemist who could eliminate it.

Whether you believe cellulite is just plain body fat or a special version of trapped and toxic fat, you may have fallen for the lure of creams, lotions, sweat devices, and rollers that attempt to trim it from your body.

Creams and lotions are effective only for smoothing the texture of the skin and slightly diminishing the cottage-cheese look, but they work only as long as you apply them. Liposuction is good for removing fat stores, but it can sometimes leave loose, sagging skin with dimples if you don't follow the after-surgery protocol for recovery.

A new procedure called endermologie attempts to reduce the appearance of cellulite with a combination of external suction through a computer-controlled machine and vigorous massage by trained medical personnel. The procedure works on the fibrous connections, making them more flexible so that there is less dimpling and anchoring of skin to the underlying muscle. Good candidates are people with small areas of irregular fat who do not want a surgical procedure. Of course, people who part with the time and cash for this procedure should maximize their chances by enjoying daily physical activity, drinking more fluids, and reducing fat intake in general. They also shouldn't be surprised if the positive results are only temporary.

▶ Diets

You've heard that they don't work, yet, if you're like most people, you may still be tempted to try every fad diet that comes along. Whether they're high-protein or all-grapefruit, fad diets are dangerous because they eliminate three basic principles of good nutrition: moderation, variety, and balance. It may sound trite, but eating a nutritious diet and increasing exercise (with twice as much strength training as aerobics) is still the best way to build lean muscle mass, which is your primary fat-burning engine.

The reality is that some people are naturally lean no matter how much they eat, and others seem to gain weight just by eyeing dessert. Thus, if you're dealing with comparable lifestyles, the reason that one guy is heavy and his pal is skinny hinges on one undeniable factor: metabolism. That's why, in addition to a sensible eating plan and plenty of activity, supplements that help you increase muscle mass, such as l-carnitine (as long as you're exercising), and herbs such as *Garcinia cambogia* and ephedra (also known as ma huang) can be helpful.

Don't count on calorie-reduction diets to keep added pounds off you for the long term. Loads of scientific evidence now indicates that your body will adjust to any temporary loss with an upward adjustment that usually surpasses the original weight.

As for increasing protein intake to 40 percent of calories (with 30 percent from carbohydrates and 30 percent from fat), as some new diets recommend, or adding more fiber to your diet, I find there is plenty of anecdotal evidence to support claims that these measures have prevented further weight gain. I think their real merit is based on replacing some empty calories (sweets, fats, and junk foods) with healthier foods.

➤ Glucosamine Sulfate

I couldn't recommend daily, hourly movement without also addressing the facts that we're an aging population and that moving in general may not be as comfortable as it once was. As we age, changes occur in our joints. Normal wear and tear on cartilage and synovial capsules (lubricated enclosures that protect your joints and keep the bones from grinding against each other) can lead to increased stiffness, inflexibility, and minor aches and pains.

On top of that, if you've been active, perhaps as a runner or skier, you may have had a few spills mixed in with your thrills. That usually means a sore knee, an aching back, or an occasional "trick" ankle. Whatever the nagging complaints, aging generally shows up in our joints first, and I predict that during the next several years, we are going to see a wave of products and remedies for eliminating the distress of growing old "before our time." I want to share with you a few tricks of the nutrient trade to keep your joints in prime condition.

The chief one is glucosamine sulfate, a naturally occurring substance normally formed from glucose and found in high concentrations in joint structures. When it is taken up by joint tissues, glucosamine exerts a powerful therapeutic effect. In more than 300 scientific investigations and more than 20 double-blind, placebo-controlled studies, it has been shown to be virtually free of side effects. If you have the first stages of osteoarthritis, glucosamine can help alleviate any painful symptoms and has been proven to be better tolerated than ibuprofen. That means no gastrointestinal upset, heartburn, or nausea.

How many of us practically kiss the bottles of nonsteroidal anti-inflammatory drugs (NSAIDs) such as ibuprofen and naproxen when we're in pain? They seem like wonder drugs, don't they? These drugs mask pain so well that you wonder if you're still injured.

There's a high price for that kind of blanket pain relief, however. In the long run, NSAIDs are toxic to your kidneys and liver and cause stomach upset, headaches, dizziness, and long-term damage to bones and cartilage by actually altering metabolism. The clear advantage of a natural compound such as glucosamine is that it provides long-term treatment of the arthritic condition, prevents further breakdown of the cartilage, and regenerates new joint tissue, including cartilage.

If you've fallen in love with your walking routine but have to cope with nagging aches in your back, knees, hips, or ankle joints, consider fortifying your cartilage, skeletal muscles, and tendons with glucosamine sulfate and other supplements, such as a combination of calcium and magnesium.

➤ Hormones

If they were good for one stage of life, they're good for all stages, right? Wrong. What has happened to common sense? Millions of people are taking hormone supplements that have not been sufficiently tested for effectiveness and safety throughout the life span. For many hormones, the jury is still out regarding long-term side effects.

Longevity seekers are convinced that supplements and medically supervised injections of human growth hormone will help reverse the aging process. The Longevity Fitness Clinic, an outpatient medical consulting service in Glendale, California, that specializes in restoring youthful vigor to aging clients, administers injections of growth hormone to people whose blood tests show that they are deficient. Growth hormone surges in youngsters, who are busy growing bones and other tissues. After that, the levels naturally taper off—and it's this "deficiency" that the injections are purported to treat. It's still not completely clear what long-term side effects may occur from taking growth hormone once we're past the age of rapid growth. The Food and Drug Administration (FDA) has made over-the-counter growth hormone illegal, although it's sold in Europe.

Another hormone, melatonin, has been the subject of more than 200 well-documented studies. Babies have the highest percentage of circulating melatonin, which is part of the reason that they sleep "like babies." By age 20, the amount of melatonin produced by the body decreases by half, and by age 45, by half again. A small amount of melatonin, less than five milligrams, helps restore good sleep patterns, but the effect of larger amounts is unknown.

➤ Estrogen Replacement Therapy

Many menopausal women consider this therapy to ease the discomfort of hot flashes and vaginal dryness. Most important, however, they consider taking it to reduce the risk of a number of degenerative conditions, including heart disease, osteoporosis, and possibly Alzheimer's disease. The standard estrogen drug prescribed for women in the United States is Premarin (derived from the urine of pregnant mares); it is often combined with progesterone.

If menopausal women want to reduce serious health risks by replacing the hormones that their bodies once produced naturally, I can understand and support that wholeheartedly. That decision should be made by you after considering your health history—as well as your mother's and grandmothers'—and weighing all the odds with a caring health practitioner. By all means, however, replace your hormones with human hormones, not the bizarre mixture of unnatural versions that are dangerous and completely foreign to a woman's body. These mass-marketed, off-target estrogens are responsible for creating little horses, not humans. Contact a compounding pharmacist and work with a physician who understands natural hormone replacement. Don't fall for the propaganda of mega-billion-dollar pharmaceutical firms that there is nothing adverse about taking hormones derived from a pregnant horse's urine. To find a medical doctor who will prescribe natural hormones, contact the American College for Advancement in Medicine at (800) 532-3688.

➤ Intimacy

Love, romance, and mutual attraction can help you become aware of how much life matters, and suddenly you'll take better care of yourself. Compare it to a time when you were lonely or without friends to see how your habits can change for the better. Fall in love, and watch your satiety levels change as you eat. You're being nourished by another source and no longer need to stuff yourself on Saturday nights alone with *Seinfeld* reruns.

Aside from the butterflies of infatuation, love and intimacy seem to have a fundamental impact on our well-being and survival. Dean Ornish, M.D., of the Preventive Medicine Research Institute in Sausalito, California, found that 50 years ago, only 5 percent of people lived alone, compared to 25 percent today. This isolation takes a toll on many areas of a person's life, affecting diet and activity and limiting social networks of support. When you experience the healing power of love, your immune and cardiac systems operate better. Part of the reason may be that you make more healthful lifestyle choices, supported by people who care about you.

➤ Liposuction

I like it. This may be the first fitness book in history with an author willing to go on the line and admit it. When it comes to small-scale reduction of certain unwanted fatty deposits, liposuction is very effective. I had it done on saddle bags, and I've never regretted it.

People look a little shocked when I tell them this. They expect a health and fitness authority to stand before them and say "only sensible eating and daily exercise," and forget the rest. Let me clarify a couple of points.

First, I'm not against cosmetic surgery. I'm against lying about it. When people pose as perfect models for exercise but have undergone years of cosmetic lifts, tucks, and sucks, they present false images and unrealistic goals to the public.

I'm also against liposuction as a weight-loss procedure. High-volume liposuction, in which people beg surgeons to remove unhealthy amounts of fat, is dangerous. The removal of more than five liters of fat in one surgical procedure can cause a life-threatening imbalance of fluids, edema (swelling), shock, and sometimes death.

Nevertheless, if you've fretted and moaned about your double chin or chubby knees to the point of boring yourself and others, and you wish you could just get on with life, you may be a good candidate for small-volume liposuction. It's ideal for spot reducing areas of the body that do not respond well to diet and exercise alone. Remember, however, that even though liposuction will remove fat cells in that area for good, there is always the chance that you will increase the size of remaining ones by not maintaining a healthy lifestyle.

If you're considering liposuction or any other kind of plastic or cosmetic surgery, ask yourself the following questions.

Is the technique I'm considering less than five years old? Many new methods are being tested now, and some won't be here for long. Other new techniques are thriving because of marketing hype, but they aren't necessarily better. Laser surgery, for example, attempts to accomplish the same results as a scalpel but is only as effective as the surgeon using it, according to Fredric Newman, M.D., a prominent New York plastic and reconstructive surgeon. The bottom line is, don't let yourself become a test subject; agree only to a method that is tried and true.

Does it sound too good to be true? It probably is. You can't have a facelift in the afternoon and go to work the next morning. There are no surgeries that don't result in some temporary redness, bruising, or swelling.

Am I hoping for a better life afterward? Don't bet on it. Stay realistic about what you're purchasing: an altered appearance. Also, sometimes the reality of the alteration is not what you had in mind and will take some emotional adjustment. This is not for those who are beset with perfectionism. Discuss every aspect of what the procedure entails with a board-certified, highly recommended plastic surgeon and his staff. Most important, realize that you will have the same life as you always did. Plastic surgery will not create a new romance, give your life meaning and purpose, or make you happy. It will simply give you a new appearance.

➤ Longevity Elixirs

I'm completely reluctant to take any of the anti-aging cocktails that are being dreamt up in the longevity research labs today. We simply don't know the long-term effects of taking supplemental human growth hormone, DHEA, and other "anti-aging" products.

We do know the long-term effects of our expectations, however. One of my favorite studies found that the most consistent measure of someone's longevity turns out to be not genetics, lifestyle, or diet, but expectations. When researchers asked people, "How long do you expect to live?" they discovered that people who imagined 50 years lived until then, and people who foresaw a life into their nineties were pretty close to that. If that's the case, you'd better adjust your life expectancy attitude to fit your goals.

In the meantime, follow this recipe for living longer from the MacArthur Foundation, a private institution based in Chicago that funds studies on human health and longevity.

- Keep blood pressure under 140/90 mmHg (millimeters of mercury).
- Avoid excessive use of alcohol, saturated fats, and sugars.
- Prevent disease through healthy lifestyle and early detection.
- Get lots of daily exercise, including aerobics and weight training.
- Don't smoke.
- Avoid overexposure to the sun.

In addition, there's a suspicion that eating slightly less than your body asks for (that is, going through life slightly hungry rather than contentedly full) may do for humans what it does for every species of animal tested—help them live longer, healthier lives.

➤ Massage

The healing powers of massage are evident to anyone who has benefited from a skilled bodyworker's attention. Now it appears that massage is not just great for relaxing tension and soothing muscles but also for boosting the immune system and helping babies grow.

The therapeutic value of massage has been investigated under several National Institutes of Health grants during the past few years, and it continues to be hailed as a revolution in gentle, noninvasive health care, capable of saving billions of dollars in health-care costs each year.

Studies have shown that levels of immunoglobulin A, an infection-fighting protein, climb rapidly following a massage. Also, in studies with premature and low-birthweight babies, the infants who received daily massage grew twice as fast as those who were not massaged. Surgical patients heal more rapidly. Anxiety, depression, and headaches take less of a toll, and workers' productivity and sense of well-being are absolutely enhanced.

In fact, massage is crucial for alleviating the severe back pain and poor posture that result from hunching over computers and workstations.

Instead of a five-minute coffee break, workers who took a five-minute break for a massage, especially on the head, neck, and shoulder tension zone—

what I call the Bermuda Triangle of stress—were able to go back to their jobs with more creativity and accuracy, according to studies.

You can learn how to give and receive a basic massage by watching the video "Esalen Massage," the first follow-along video program from the world-famous Esalen Institute, a leader in mind/body exploration and experimental education. Write to the Esalen Institute, Highway 1, Big Sur, CA 93920-9616.

➤ Natural Progesterone

I'm placing this under "natural" rather than "progesterone" to emphasize the difference. The most widely prescribed progesterone for postmenopausal women in the United States is medroxyprogesterone acetate (MPA). It's prescribed in combination with estrogen in the hope that it will prevent the rise in uterine cancer risk experienced by women who receive estrogen replacement alone. New studies, however, indicate that MPA may cut off coronary blood flow, leading to a higher heart attack rate.

Women in the studies on natural progesterone did fine. You can find it in topical creams such as Mexican yam cream. Be sure to look for "progesterone," not "progestin," on the ingredients list.

➤ Pyruvate

I've looked at all the studies on this nutrient, and I can understand why people are frustrated if they take pyruvate supplements for weight loss and never lose a pound. It only seems to help with fat-burning in half the people who take it, half of the time. In studies, the differences in weight loss between placebo groups (with healthy diets and similar exercise schedules but no pyruvate supplements) and the supplement groups are only a matter of a pound or two. I wouldn't waste my money on it.

➤ Thermogenic Agents

Thermogenesis is your ability to produce heat for warmth by burning calories from food and sometimes from body fat. One way that we create thermogenesis is by shivering. A more efficient way to warm the internal organs is accomplished by brown adipose tissue (BAT), a form of fat that is specifically designed to convert calories into heat energy. You store brown fat mostly around your heart and lungs, with a little around your intestines. As a baby, you have a lot, but the supply decreases with age.

People with very active brown fat have a sort of free ticket in life. It seems that they are able to burn off excess calories and therefore can eat whatever they want. They're also the types of people who feel overheated after eating a big meal.

On the other hand, people who tend to gain weight easily are often chilly. Their BAT stores are not functioning as actively. However, when these folks take their first thermogenic product such as ephedra or caffeine, they not only experience warm sensations for the first time ("I actually kicked off the covers when sleeping!"), they begin to convert some white fat (the stuff you can pinch) into fuel for their brown fat cells. They begin to burn fat like a normally lean person. That makes thermogenic products seem like miracles.

With an appetite-suppression product such as Dexatrim, however, there is a price to pay. Since it includes phenylpropanolamine, a huge toll is placed on the body and its hormonal system. Furthermore, because metabolic stimulation of brown fat has a direct effect on your nervous sytem, many products are not recommended for pregnant or nursing women; people with heart disease, high blood pressure, or thyroid conditions; or anyone who is taking prescription medications or has other medical limitations.

Herbal compounds are safer alternatives. They start with the plant ephedra (not synthetic ephedrine) and blend it with about a dozen other herbs and nutrients to balance the stimulating effect. I've talked with thousands of people who have successfully managed to boost their metabolic burn and lose body fat with these products. Unfortunately, ephedra has been attacked by the media for being unsafe, based on completely unreliable statistics. I have investigated ephedra, and I discovered that the harsh claims were grossly overstated, particularly when the herb was used at the recommended dosages.

I'm often asked about weight-loss products that contain synthetic ephedrine instead of whole ephedra. You're always better off with a whole plant working in harmony with other balanced and stimulating herbs. Without that synergy, you simply have the intensive effects of any synthetic component—plenty of "buzz" and overstimulation, but no effective brown fat stimulation.

► **Wars (False Ones)**

Pardon me while I bow out of the latest war on fat. Just like the war on drugs and the war on poverty, this latest crusade is distasteful in its rhetoric, lacking in understanding and compassion, and beset with a medical arrogance that ensures that there will never be a peaceful surrender, let alone a victorious conclusion. It's a collection of misguided misinformation missiles, aimed at hurting the folks it is seemingly meant to help.

We know beyond a doubt that long-term nonsurgical treatment of obesity in adults is largely unsuccessful, no matter whether the focus is dietary guidelines, physical activity, behavior modification programs, diet clinics, or diet drugs. Also, there are numerous surveys that show that at least 95 percent of people who enter weight-loss programs regain the lost weight within two to five years.

Instead of declaring war, fall in love. Reframe your situation by loving your body into better condition. One study showed that restrictive diets don't keep people at their healthy weights, but taking a class to boost self-esteem had a lasting effect on weight loss.

SORTING THROUGH SUPPLEMENT HYPE

Some of our most deadly and disabling diseases could be prevented with regular use of nutritional supplements. According to David Heber, M.D., Ph.D., director of the University of California, Los Angeles, Center for Human Nutrition, "We now have a substantial body of data showing that if everyone took a few supplements every day, they could significantly lower their risk of a multitude of serious diseases."

Every year, you hear about a supplement that the public should have taken but didn't because of the reluctance of government dietary agencies, the Food and Drug Administration, and so-called nutritional experts to depart from the tried-and-true advice, "just eat a balanced diet, and you won't have to worry." You hear about how the birth defect spina bifida can be prevented with a simple daily supplement of 400 micrograms of folic acid. Or how B-complex vitamins can lower homocysteine levels and possibly reduce heart attacks. Or how early daily supplementation with 1,200 milligrams of calcium, 400 international units of vitamin D, and at least 500 milligrams of magnesium can reduce the risk of osteoporosis and potentially prevent 50,000 hip fractures annually.

As a journalist, I've talked to laboratory scientists doing tests on vitamin E, and I found out that they've been taking at least 400 international units daily for several years to prevent heart disease, cancer, and other diseases. They didn't wait for the big bureaucratic wheels of government agencies to update the national guidelines.

Also, according to a New Jersey study, infectious diseases in the elderly can be reduced by strengthening the immune system with a daily multivitamin.

So, yes, I'm a big advocate of nutritional supplements for a healthier life. If you were to plot out a 1-to-10 scale, with 1 being "just get your vitamins from food" and 10 standing for total supplement mania—swallowing every nutritional supplement available—I'm right around a 6 or 7. The following are my personal favorites. Create a supplement cabinet in your kitchen based on your own health-risk profile.

➤ B-Complex Vitamins

Researchers in Sweden and Norway are way ahead of the United States in outlining the importance of B-complex vitamins. They found that low blood levels of B_6, niacin, and folate (the naturally occurring form of folic acid) led to high levels of homocysteine, a by-product of protein metabolism that can damage arteries, and that excess homocysteine is a strong predictor of death from coronary artery disease.

➤ Calcium

Calcium is important for strong skeletons, healthy teeth, and myriad cellular and muscular actions, yet half of all American children do not get the recommended amount of calcium, and many adults are falling short, too. Try to get 1,000 to 1,200 milligrams a day from foods such as leafy greens, cheese, yogurt, broccoli, and fat-free milk. Then consider taking a calcium supplement.

Citrate formulations are expensive but may be worth the extra cost if you don't absorb other calcium supplements well. To keep your body's mineral levels in balance, combine your calcium supplement with an equal or slightly lower dose of magnesium.

➤ Carnitine

Found mostly in red meat, this amino acid helps transport fats for energy metabolism. People who haven't exercised for a while and are out of shape benefit most from l-carnitine tartrate. There's a lot of anecdotal evidence that 500 to 1,000 milligrams a day of carnitine will increase fat loss when combined with a low-carbohydrate diet. Most of the scientific studies done on carnitine have focused on athletic endurance, however, and showed significant improvement.

➤ Coenzyme Q$_{10}$

This substance acts like an antioxidant, destroying the unstable molecules called free radicals that can damage cells. At doses of 60 milligrams daily, coenzyme Q$_{10}$ becomes a booster for proper function of the mitochondria, a cell's energy powerhouse, which in turn protects against heart disease. As more and more study results are revealed, we may hear of more benefits from this supplement.

➤ Creatine

Like carnitine, creatine monohydrate has long been popular with athletes and bodybuilders, but until recently, there hasn't been much support from scientists. The American College of Sports Medicine reports that creatine helped athletes gain in lean muscle mass, lifting performance, and sprinting speed. Research has also found that taking creatine supplements can increase levels of HDL, the good cholesterol. Researchers at the University of Memphis warn, however, that the medical safety of prolonged creatine supplementation hasn't been determined yet.

➤ Echinacea

Keep a liquid extract of this herb on hand. European studies show that it's helpful as a natural immunity booster during infections. Taking it early and often during the first stages of a cold or flu can diminish the symptoms.

➤ Essential Fatty Acids

Omega-3 fish oils are a daily staple for me. Taking just 13 grams a day will reduce the risk of cardiovascular disease, improve mental and visual functions, and ease PMS symptoms. Fish oils, from tuna and other large ocean fish, contain essential fatty acids such as docosahexaenoic acid (DHA) and eicosapentaenoic acid (EPA). Conjugated linoleic acid (CLA), found in cheese and meat products, may promote development of lean muscle and burn fat more effectively.

For the past 20 years, we've been taught that fat is the ultimate diet demon, but not all fats are culprits. You should avoid unhealthy fats (hydrogenated and partially hydrogenated fats, animal fats, and oxidized trans fats in margarine), but including the right kind of essential fatty acids and some monounsaturated fats such as olive oil is crucial for overall health, the immune system, and appetite satisfaction.

➤ Evening Primrose Oil

This oil is a source of gamma-linolenic acid, or GLA. It soothes PMS symptoms and is helpful in reducing high blood pressure, relieving rheumatoid arthritis pain, lowering high cholesterol, and treating diabetic neuropathy, the nerve damage that can result from diabetes. Look for a supplement that contains at least 500 milligrams of GLA.

➤ Fiber

Think of the two types of fiber—soluble and insoluble—as the sponge and the sweeper. We need them both, yet few people get sufficient amounts of either. Soluble fiber (such as oat bran, pectin, and beans and other legumes) sponges up wastes and toxins, lowers blood fats, reduces the risk of heart disease and stroke, and stabilizes blood sugar. Insoluble fiber (such as whole grains, high-fiber vegetables, and psyllium) helps with weight loss by making you feel full, promotes regularity, and may help lower colorectal cancer risk. Remember, though, that whenever you increase your fiber intake, you need to increase your water intake, too.

➤ 5-HTP

Michael Murray, N.D., a naturopathic doctor and co-author of *The Encyclopedia of Natural Medicine*, swears by this supplement, and that's good enough for me. A naturally occurring neurochemical, 5-HTP is a precursor of serotonin, the neurotransmitter that affects mood, sleep, appetite, sex, and other body functions.

➤ Flaxseed Oil

This oil is another good source of omega-3's, the essential fatty acids that are good for immunity, metabolism, and the proper functioning of many systems. You can buy bottles of it in health food stores and use it in recipes.

➤ Folic Acid

You need 400 micrograms a day of this B vitamin if you're of child-bearing age, and this amount is next to impossible to get from foods alone. Folic acid prevents certain birth defects. It's also a protective agent in lowering homocysteine levels as a cardiac risk factor and in reducing the risk of some cancers.

➤ Ginkgo Biloba

This herb seems to improve blood flow and brain circulation and therefore may be excellent for mental functioning, possibly preventing Alzheimer's disease and memory loss. It's been called a "memory enhancer and brain food" in medical journals.

➤ Ginseng

Valued for thousands of years in Asia as a longevity aid, ginseng may boost performance and prevent fatigue and chronic disease.

➤ Green Tea

More popular in Asia than the black teas Americans normally drink, the green version has more catechins, which neutralize free radicals and reduce your risk of cancer. Drink a cup a day.

➤ Phytonutrients

These are naturally occurring nutrients found in fruits and vegetables that protect against heart disease and cancer and help boost immunity. Although the recommendation is to eat five to nine servings of fruits and vegetables a day, most of us don't eat anywhere near that amount. Until you join the ranks of the rare 10 percent who do eat the recommended amounts, take a phytonutrient supplement.

➤ Probiotics

Not all bacteria are bad for you. In particular, your intestines need certain bacteria to digest food. Sometimes, however, these "friendly" bacteria lose their dominance to an overgrowth of unhealthy flora, parasites, bad bacteria, and candida (yeast). This can cause short-term distress, but it also may well be the basis of many chronic conditions, such as fibromyalgia and chronic fatigue syndrome. If you experience excessive bloating, gas, indigestion, and sugar cravings, you probably need to restore normal bowel bacteria. Probiotics, which are supplements that propagate good bacteria, can help achieve that. Take a high-potency probiotic formula that contains both acidophilus and bifidobacteria.

➤ St. John's Wort

This mood-lifting botanical works well for mild depression, but do not take it if you're taking prescription antidepressants.

➤ Saw Palmetto Berry

This herb is important for men because it helps treat benign prostatic hyperplasia, a bunch of big words that mean a swollen prostate. Saw palmetto will alter the results of a prostate specific antigen, or PSA, test, which is used to detect prostate cancer, so be sure to tell your physician if you're taking it.

➤ Selenium

This important antioxidant mineral may prevent some cancers and may also be helpful in protecting against heart disease. Take 500 micrograms or less a day.

➤ Vitamin C

An excellent antioxidant that protects against cancer, heart disease, diabetes, and cataract formation, vitamin C may also help reduce cold symptoms. Most people need at least 250 milligrams a day, according to experts. People who have diabetes should take 1,200 milligrams twice daily, according to Len Saputo, M.D., director of Health Medicine Forum.

➤ Vitamin E

Due to the overwhelming evidence that it's a protective antioxidant that fights cancer, heart disease, and other degenerative conditions, this is the supplement that's probably most swallowed by laboratory researchers. You must take at least 400 international units daily to reap these protective effects. If you are taking anticoagulants (blood thinners), though, check with your doctor first.

➤ Zinc

This mineral is necessary for proper organ and hormone functioning. Men need it for prostate health, and pregnant women who take a multivitamin with zinc can reduce the chance of their babies being born at low birthweights.

Unleashing
Your Seventh Sense

You've reached the end of *The Fitness Instinct,* but you're actually just beginning your journey to instinctual fitness.

Now you're ready to move as you've never moved before. Once you've firmly tapped into your fitness instinct, you'll start to love movement. Yes, you'll become more fit. But that's just a by-product, a result of tapping into the desire to move that was buried inside for years, just yearning to get out.

During your journey, you may relapse. That's normal. You may catch yourself yearning for a tighter body or forcing yourself to stay on the stair-stepper or vegetating in front of the tube. Don't beat yourself up. When you relapse, just take a refresher course and brush up on what you've learned in this book.

- Movement personality. Take the self-tests again, and continue to do so throughout your lifetime. You may find that as you grow and change, so will your movement personality. Connect to what's authentically you: Racer, Stroller, Dancer, or Trekker. Keep tailoring fitness activities to suit your unique self.
- MythFits. Detach from an image-oriented culture and a cult of perfection. Forget a lot of what you've been taught about the "right" way to exercise. Transfer authority back within you.
- Positive thinking. Stop the negative body talk and replace it with words that inspire daily, life-enhancing movement.

- Take-charge attitude. Remember, you're not doing this for your doctor, spouse, mother, or friends. You're doing it for you. Recognize that you're the one in charge of your physical self.
- Still point. Do some deep breathing. Try a visualization. Meditate. It's the ultimate paradox in our hurry-up society, but you have to pause before you go.
- Seventh sense. Remember those inborn instincts. Do your body scan. Sense when your body wants to move, stretch, play, jump, tumble, wiggle, rest, and dance as if nobody's watching. Assess your physical state: tired, wired, mired, or uninspired. Determine what your body needs in the moment: an energy generator, de-stressing soother, moveable treat, or creative spark.
- Circadian rhythms. Make sure that your exercise choices match up with your energy cycles, which fluctuate from dawn through daytime and dusk.
- Inspiration. Link your movement choices to what inspires you most: beauty, information, courage, or comfort.
- Gathering 30. Remember, you don't have to make a marathon out of this. A brisk 5-minute walk may be all your body needs right now. Just gather 30 minutes of movement as you go about your day.
- Alternative moves. As time marches on, so will they. Continue to experiment with new classes. You'll be surprised by what you positively enjoy.
- Core desire. Don't beat yourself up for lacking motivation. Let it be born of fiery passion. Review which core desire is operating at full tilt at any one time and be happy in serving it.

CREATE YOUR OWN LIFE DANCE

You now have a myriad of playful recipes for practicing holistic fitness. In a sense, you are creating your unique life dance, a signature of rhythm, movement, and flow. Eventually, moving every hour will be almost second nature to you. In fact, within a few weeks, you will notice how much more supple, vigorous, and alert your entire body seems. You'll notice how you bring your life dance into every situation, from quieter moments to stress-filled times. Your dance and your breath will be your strongest allies for peace of mind and well-being.

Good luck with all the techniques in this book. They are meant to help you grow in heightened mind-body awareness, enjoying activities that are most meaningful to you. The path to fitness is ultimately a spiritual journey, rich in self-discovery. Above all, I hope that you have a new appreciation for movement, to the point where it becomes an irrepressible daily act. As you transform your thinking about exercise and replace it with a passion to move for the pure joy of it, you will also transform your relationship with your body. From a baby's first steps to a 50th anniversary waltz, movement softens time's relentless passage with a beguiling rhythm.

Opening to your natural instinct to move, the powerful life force within you, may be the most intimate and supportive way to spend time with yourself. Enjoy all of the alternative fitness paths, from heart-stirring creative sparks to soft-landing soothers. May all of your experiences be moving, and may your fitness instinct stay alive and well!

index

F

about the author

For nearly three decades, Peg Jordan has been a tireless researcher, journalist, trainer, and speaker in the fields of fitness and health. Currently, Jordan is editor-in-chief of *American Fitness* magazine, the official publication of the Aerobics and Fitness Association of America. She is a frequent guest commentator for NBC-TV's *The Today Show* and for CNN; she is the Fitness and Wellness expert for ivillage.com, the number one women's network site on the Web; and she is regularly consigned to write articles and commentaries for national media outlets. In addition, much of her time is spent giving speeches and seminars for organizations ranging from AT&T and Lucent Technologies to the American Heart Association and the National Fitness Leaders Association. More than 100,000 people have heard her speak in person on such topics as the fitness instinct, alternative healing, and wellness.

Jordan launched her health career as a registered nurse. In the 1980s, she served as a scriptwriter and consultant on fitness videos and infomercials for such celebrities as Cher, Kathy Smith, and Richard Simmons. For her contributions to the fitness industry, Jordan has been awarded the Healthy American Fitness Leader Award.

Jordan offers seminars and multimedia workshops on the fitness instinct, the four movement personalities, and overall healthy living. For information, contact Health and Lifestyle at (510) 482-4440, or send e-mail to jordan@flashtrends.com.